Holistic Practice in Healthcare

Holistic Practice in Healthcare

SECOND EDITION

The Burford NDU Person-centred Model

EDITED BY

Christopher Johns

Freelance Consultant, Emeritus Professor of Nursing

University of Bedfordshire, Redruth, Cornwall, UK

Forewords by Jean Watson and Brendan McCormack

WILEY Blackwell

This second edition first published 2024

Edition History
John Wiley & Sons Ltd (1e, 1994)

Registered offices
John Wiley & Sons, Inc., 111 River Street, Hoboken, NJ 07030, USA
John Wiley & Sons Ltd, The Atrium, Southern Gate, Chichester, West Sussex, PO19 8SQ, UK

For details of our global editorial offices, customer services, and more information about Wiley products visit us at www.wiley.com.

Wiley also publishes its books in a variety of electronic formats and by print-on-demand. Some content that appears in standard print versions of this book may not be available in other formats.

Library of Congress Cataloging-in-Publication Data
Names: Johns, Christopher, editor.
Title: Holistic practice in healthcare : the Burford NDU person-centred model / edited by Christopher Johns.
Other titles: Burford NDU model.
Description: Second edition. | Hoboken, NJ : Wiley-Blackwell, 2024. | Preceded by The Burford NDU model : caring in practice / edited by Christopher Johns. 1994. | Includes bibliographical references and index.
Identifiers: LCCN 2023025501 | ISBN 9781394194711 (paperback) | ISBN 9781394194742 (ebook) | ISBN 9781394194735 (epub) | ISBN 9781394194728 (pdf)
Subjects: MESH: Holistic Nursing--methods | Models, Nursing | Patient-Centered Care | Philosophy, Nursing
Classification: LCC RT84.5 | NLM WY 86.5 | DDC 610.7301--dc23/eng/20230527
LC record available at https://lccn.loc.gov/2023025501

Cover Image: © HAKKI ARSLAN/Shutterstock
Cover Design: Wiley

Set in 9.5/12.5pt STIXTwoText by Integra Software Services Pvt. Ltd, Pondicherry, India

Contents

PART 2 Practitioner Accounts

List of Contributors

Christopher Johns RN, PhD, HSGAHN was general manager of Buford hospital, Head of Buford Nursing Development Unit and Lecturer-practitioner with Oxford Brookes University between January 1989 and December 1991. It was an extremely formative period that set the tone and scope for his subsequent academic life. Now retired from Professor of nursing at the University of Bedfordshire, he maintains an active advocate of holistic and reflective practice through writing and consultation. His book *Becoming a Reflective Practitioner* is now in its sixth edition. I developed 'Reflexive narrative as self-inquiry towards self-transformation' as an approach to research published by Sage in 2017. This approach formed the core of a Masters in healthcare leadership leading to the publication of *Mindful Leadership* by Palgrave in 2015. His theories of practice have been inductively and reflexively developed informed by extant theory.

The following contributors are presented as per the 1994 text:

Susan Booker RGN ONC, Primary nurse/team leader, Oxford Community hospital.

Kate Butcher BA (Hons), RGN, Associate nurse, Ward 7e NDU, Oxford Radcliffe hospital (formerly primary nurse at Buford Community hospital).

Roger Cowell, BA, RGN, Primary nurse, Buford Community hospital.

Robert Garbett, RGN, BN(Hons), Project worker/ team leader, Ward 7e NDU, Oxford Radcliffe hospital.

Carol McCaffrey, Fourth year student BA (Hons) nursing programme at Oxford Brookes University.

Susan Metcalf, SRN, SCM, NDU, Cert, CPT District nurse and clinical practice teacher.

Lyn Sutherland RGN, ITU Cert., Dip.HE (DN) District nurse, Jericho Health Centre Oxford (formerly primary nurse at Buford Community hospital).

To Jean Watson, PhD, RN, AHN-BC, FAAN, LL (AAN) is Distinguished Professor and Dean Emerita, University of Colorado Denver, College of Nursing Anschutz Medical Center campus, where she held the nation's first endowed Chair in Caring Science for 16 years. She is founder of the original Center for Human Caring in Colorado and is a Fellow of the American Academy of Nursing; past President of the National League for Nursing; founding member of International Association in Human Caring and International Caritas Consortium. She is Founder and Director of the non-profit foundation, Watson Caring Science Institute (www.watsoncaringscience.org). In 2013 Dr. Watson was inducted as a Living Legend by the American Academy of Nursing, its highest honour.

She is a widely published author and recipient of many national/international awards and honours, including: The Fetzer Institute Norman Cousins Award, in recognition of her commitment to developing; maintaining and exemplifying relationship-centred care practices; an international Kellogg Fellowship in Australia; a Fulbright Research Award in Sweden; The Hildebrand Center for Compassion in Medicine Award Notre Dame University; Academy Integrative Medicine and Healing Award for pioneering work in Caring Science; Japanese International Society of Caring and Peace Chair. She holds sixteen (16) Honorary Doctoral Degrees, including 13 International Honorary Doctorates (E. G. Sweden, United Kingdom, Spain, British Colombia and Quebec, Canada, Japan, Turkey, Peru and Colombia, S. America, Ireland).

Dr. Watson's caring philosophy and Transpersonal Theory of Human Caring, and Caritas Processes of Caring Science are used to guide transformative models of caring education; and professional caring- healing practices for hospitals, nurses and patients alike, in diverse settings worldwide.

As author /co-author of over 30 books on caring, her latest books range from empirical measurements and international research on caring, mindful caring science practices, to new postmodern philosophies of caring and healing, philosophy and science of caring and caring science as sacred science and global advance in caring literacy. Her books have been AJN books of the year awards and seek to bridge paradigms as well as point towards transformative models for this 21st century.

To Professor Brendan McCormack D.Phil (Oxon.), BSc (Hons.), FRCN, FEANS, FRCSI, PGCEA, RMN, RGN, FAAN, MAE is Head of The Susan Wakil School of Nursing and Midwifery (inc. Sydney Nursing School) and Dean, Faculty of Medicine and Health, The University of Sydney; Extraordinary Professor, Department of Nursing, University of Pretoria, South Africa; Professor of Nursing, Maribor University, Slovenia; Visiting Professor, Ulster University; Adjunct Professor, Zealand University Hospital/University of Southern Denmark; Professor II, Østfold University College, Norway; Professor of Nursing, Queen Margaret University, Edinburgh.

Brendan's research focuses on person-centredness with a particular focus on the development of person-centred cultures, practices and processes. He has engaged in this work at all levels from theory development to implementation science and through to instrument design, testing and evaluation. He is methodologically diverse, but is most at home in participatory/action research. Whilst he has a particular expertise in gerontology and dementia practices, his work has spanned all specialities and is multi-professional. He also has a particular focus on the use of arts and creativity in healthcare research and development. Brendan has more than 600 published outputs, including 240 peer-reviewed publications in international journals and 12 books. Brendan is a Fellow of The European Academy of Nursing Science, Fellow of the Royal College of Nursing, Fellow of the Royal College of Surgeons in Ireland and Fellow of the American Academy of Nursing. In 2014 he was awarded the 'International Nurse Researcher Hall of Fame' by Sigma Theta Tau International. Most recently, Brendan was featured in the Wiley Publishers 'Inspiring Minds' short films series https://www.youtube.com/watch?v=13c5C-tbcT4. In 2022 Brendan was selected as a member of The Academia Europaea.

Foreword by Jean Watson

Jean Watson, PhD, RN, AHN-BC, FAAN, LL (AAN)

From decade to decade, from one century to another, hospitals and healthcare systems have grappled with Nursing and Nurses. Now, each are faced with even greater upheavals with Post-COVID survival, as our industrialized healthcare institutions are turning upside down, and inside out.

Outdated industrial, economically dominated healthcare mindsets are now having to face loss of core values, meaning, and purpose; resulting in loss of nurses, dispirited nurses, shortage of nurses, turnover of nurses, retention of nurses, unhappy nurses, 'less resilient' nurses and on it goes. In their own way, each are grasping at short-term straws for any superficial 'fix it' tactic to solve this looming, but longstanding institutional human care, nursing quandary.

There is open critique from the public, worldwide, that continues from one decade, one century to another, that the so-called modern, healthcare industry is really a sick-care, body-physical, techno cure system – a system built upon an industrial, product model which differentiated diagnosis, technical treatments from patient/family personal meaning. A system that separated human from their humanity, their culture, spirituality, beliefs, and inner life world of subjectivity, in relation to outcomes. This dominant medicalized, institutional method of control over humanity has reigned over nurses and patients alike. It has been void of self-control, self-knowledge, self-care, self-choices for health and self-healing.

The result: Nursing being restricted from practicing its own profession. Nursing being restricted from its core values, philosophical moral, ethical covenant with humanity and human caring/healing/health for all. Such an industrial model, dominates, to this day, even while knowing other options. Without attention to the evolved, spirit-filled paradigm of health and human caring/healing that integrates nursing's foundational disciplinary philosophy and core values, the inevitable conclusion is that Nurses and hospitals, can no longer endure outdated, detached, medicalized, clinicalized, 'doing' models.

In mainstream organizations, there ironically remains, a proclivity for a dominant practice pattern, disconnecting one's theory and disciplinary grounding about the nature of nursing and nature of human experiences. Thus, there is reluctance to give voice, language, and informed reflection and critique to guide one's actions. Nurses at bedside often left with inability to articulate Nursing to self/system and the public.

To this day, the discourse from within nursing itself, including the American Academy of Nursing, and American Association of Colleges of Nursing continue to debate in despair how to address the 'nursing workforce shortage', the critical need for nurses (al la bodies) to serve a dysfunctional sick-care system of hospitals, in contrast to maturing professional nursing. Beyond hospital nursing culture and patterns. (Author, AAN program, 2022).

In spite of knowing better, mainstream nursing education and practices continue to have an affinity, almost a bias, towards focus on functional, concrete tasks institutional technical skills. This focused mentality is geared towards satisfying the technical accountability demands of a dysfunctional medical, institutional bureaucracy. In turn, restricting and limiting new patterns of professional practice to improve outdated systems, promoting hospital nurses to be directly accountable to the public for caring, healing, health. As such, nursing's caring ethos has been eclipsed from its natural prominence and place in the conventional medical-care system.

Moreover, the overriding culture of the patriarchal system, in spite of new societal awakenings for equity, diversity, and inclusivity, continues to further restrict nursing from its full development as a distinct discipline, within both practice and academic settings.

Ironically, in midst of these perennial institutional, historic and contemporary Nursing impasses, a timeless global model from the mid-eighties existed within our sight, but oddly overlooked, passed by, and out of sight. Christopher John's revised edition of the UK Burford Nursing Development, Professional Practice model, uncovers solutions to status quo institutional thinking.

It offers up a powerful mature Professional Nursing model of human caring/healing and health; grounded and informed by and from Nursing's own disciplinary solutions, overturning solidified institutional cultures. In this pre/postmodern world of medical science despair, and disorder of our human-environment healthcare/body physical, materialistic, technological 'sick care' system, there is overwhelming agreement that nursing education and healthcare are in a state of post-COVID disequilibrium. As a result, the institutional, scientific, and technological orientation of today's medical and nursing care systems cannot be sustained. Continuous inter/national studies and commissions, reports and research around the world indicate a growing consensus between and among the public and the nursing, medical and health community, search for dire measures to disrupt, repattern the prevailing institutionalized models. The first edition of John's book, in the eighties, demonstrated how Burford Nursing transcended the industrial depersonalized model. Even then during the eighties, the techno cure, bureaucratic hospital model was predicted as doomed, and deemed increasingly archaic and dysfunctional. The public continues to suffer the consequences. The Burford Model, in the eighties demonstrated how Nursing can offer professional caring/healing and health beyond medical/cure foci.

The original Burford model incorporated all the contemporary mandates for change; e.g. multi-disciplinary teams, broad based, integrated caring-healing practices, knowledge and skills; models that attend to praxis activities that seek to both integrate and transform the nurse's personal and professional values, beliefs, and reflective acts with clinical decision making in the concrete world of persons and individualize practices.

As John's clinical scholarship points out, 'all models of nursing are implicitly and explicitly underwritten by the assumptions of their authors concerning the nature of nursing'. It can be likewise acknowledged that all nursing practice is implicitly and explicitly influenced by the practising nurses' views and values concerning the nature of Nursing. And what it means to be human. In that nursing faces all the vicissitudes of humanity; nurses carry all the wounds of society – the joy, pain, celebrations, suffering, harms, hurts, loss, grief, death, dying, and before/beyond death/life – mystery, miracles, and unknowns. Nursing deals with paradox and ambiguity of human-universe existence.

One of the breakdowns in nursing practice is, and has been, the separation of the theories, philosophies, values, and worldview of the discipline of Nursing, from institutional professional nursing practice. The separation of one's calling, from reflective, critiquing of status quo, however, without reflective inquiry nurses has the tendency to conform and often complain, rather giving voice and informed moral action to sustain and actualize human caring-healing practices.

Without disciplinary grounding and informed reflection, critique and actions, nurses are left with inability to publicly and professionally ask new questions or constructively critique institutional care, towards generating new solutions. Solutions that overturn status quo assumptions about what matters? What counts as knowledge? Without informed disciplinary reflection nursing practice perpetuates separation of self from system; knowledge from voice; reflection from action. This non-reflective pattern tends to act without asking; tendency to conform and leap in, without stepping back, pausing, reflecting, questioning.

However, the good news is during the past four to five decades, nursing scholars and clinicians at multiple levels, behind-the-scene of conventional systems, have been questioning and revising nursing's very foundations for education, practice, and research. Such efforts have resulted in the critique of the dominant ideology of the patriarchal system; have led to the generation of multiple nursing theories, clinical nursing research, and theory-based practice models; have led to a revisiting of nursing ethics, basic philosophic beliefs, and ultimately to a re-examining of what is intended and needed for truly professional nursing practice.

For example, during the 1980s, with rise of doctoral nursing education, further important discourses emerged across developed countries about the nature of nursing science. These discourses critiqued nursing's 'modern' epistemological emphasis on empiricism, and critiqued the lack of ontological-philosophical-moral-ethical clarity and congruence among, and between ontology of 'being'; the nature of personhood, caring, health, illness and environment; and about the nature of nursing itself. This discourse brought new voice to nursing's place in healthcare; and has led to new perspectives about the nature of nursing's paradigm and the role of caring values and knowledge in theory and in practice.

Part of nursing's self-critique and revision of the profession is related to nursing coming of age, growing up as both a discipline and profession; is related to nursing gaining philosophical, moral, ontological, epistemological, and pragmatic clarity about its subject matter and its phenomena of interest, in both theory and practice.

Such critique, reflection, and study of foundational issues about nursing are related to the fact that nursing is becoming increasingly critical about its own practice. This 'becoming critical' is related to a recommitment to values and perspectives about human caring, about human-environment-caring therapeutic connections and nursing sensitive patient outcomes; is related to how basic foundational beliefs about such concepts, directly or indirectly, influence one's very acts. One's instrumental and expressive, moral and pragmatic actions in practice.

The current American Nurses Association revision of Nursing attests to new awakening, in that the profession is now catching up with the discipline. The latest (2022) ANA definition is as follows, reflecting a mature disciplinary specific paradigm for nursing's future.

> *Nursing integrates the art and science of caring and focuses on the protection, promotion, and optimization of health and human functioning; prevention of illness and injury; facilitation of healing; and alleviation of suffering through compassionate presence. Nursing is the diagnosis and treatment of human responses and advocacy in the care of individuals, families, groups, communities, and populations in recognition of the connection of all humanity. (American Nurses Association Definition of Nursing. 2022)*

Nursing's re-connection with its roots and basic values is now, at the disciplinary professional level, beginning to have an impact on the health and healing of individuals, families, and communities. At the disciplinary level, this re-connection and re-vision is allowing for a more actualized health and human caring profession to emerge for a new future, in the best tradition of Florence Nightingale. Such maturity positions nursing to truly come of age and awaken to its power to publicly and scholastically address the health challenges of these post-COVID times.

Johns' revised book on the Burford Nursing Development Unit provides a model of scholarly professional caring – healing practices, contributing to the further development of both the discipline and profession of nursing through a return to its philosophical basis for reflective caring practice and knowledge generation.

Further, the Burford model invites new innovative scholarship. It helps to explicate the details of a professional practice model that can serve as a guide and paradigm – case for transforming clinical nursing care; this revision comes as nursing seeks to respond to the public's cry for healthcare as basic human right.

Finally, as the year 2023 and beyond speeds towards us, the original Burford model is a living reminder and beacon for others who wish to challenge the critics. It offers a hopeful vision, a window of possibility for those leaders and institutions, who linger in the dominant system, but long for deep change. It brings courage and new promises for leaders and systems. It offers trust in a future for those who are fearful of the power of a mature nursing voice, which disrupt the comfort of conformity.

The Buford Community Hospital Nursing Development Model revised edition, not only reminds us of nursing's potential as a distinct health and human caring profession, but also reminds us of our social mandate to improve our reflective practice and coming of age. Calling and inviting us as humans and society to sustain Nursing's global covenant to the public now, and into our timeless, delicate, unknown human-universe future.

REFERENCES

Author. (2022). American Nurses Association. Scope and Standards of Practice. 4th Edition. ANA.

Personal Experience. (2022) American Academy of Nursing Panel. ANA Program.

Foreword by Brendan McCormack

Being Present – the 'Big Work' of Nursing Practice
Brendan McCormack

In 1994 when the Burford Nursing Development Unit (BNDU) Model of Nursing was first published I was very much at the beginning of a career in nursing that had yet to be realised. From 1991 I was employed in a unique role at the Oxford City Community Hospital that combined being a Lecturer/Practitioner with that of Clinical Lecturer in Nursing with responsibility for nursing leadership, preregistration nursing education, practice development and research. Such a role was indeed the combined vision of great nursing leaders at that time, who were passionate about the practice of nursing and ensuring that there was a synergistic relationship between the practice of nursing and the advancement of nursing knowledge. Having recently graduated with my own degree in nursing and embarking on doctoral studies, the role provided every opportunity to shape how we practised as nurses, how students experienced practice learning and how patients experienced care. No stone was left unturned in the pursuit of what I now call person-centred care and the cultures that needed to be in place to support such practices.

At the same time, Chris Johns was advancing a similar pursuit at the Burford Community Hospital in rural Oxfordshire, where one of the first nursing development units in the UK had been established by Alan Pearson. Burford was synonymous with being a testbed for nursing innovations and demonstrating the effectiveness of nursing interventions and care. It was internationally known for its work in this field and so it was 'natural' for me to connect with Chris and become part of a larger community that was concerned with nursing effectiveness, person-centredness and demonstrating the impact of nursing on the lives of people. Chris developed different models of reflective supervision that many of us who became contributors to the first edition of *The BNDU Model of Nursing* were participants in. Whilst reflection was not new to nurse education, its explicit and deliberate use as an integrated practice tool for explicating the essence of nursing, its quality and impact was new and seemed quite revolutionary at the time. At the Oxford City Community Hospital, the BNDU Model of Nursing provided us with a framework for shaping practice development and moving from a task-orientated, routinised practice model, to one that placed persons and their unique needs at the core of our focus. Bringing about such change was not easy of course and whilst most of the nursing leaders who engaged in this work bear the scars we acquired along the way, what we celebrate more often is the joy of the experience as nurse leaders, educators, researchers, and clinicians. Each of the chapters of this book reflect that joy and stand as testament to an approach to nursing that sadly feels like it was a 'unique' experience.

So twenty-eight years later, it is a humbling experience to re-read those same chapters, reflect on those practice experiences and yes, mourn what we have lost in nursing since then. In the 1994 edition of this book, Jean Watson's foreword highlighted the challenges and dilemmas for nursing at that time, as it established its evidence base, built a body of contemporary knowledge and figured out 'what matters' in practice. Watson postulated that

> *... this revision of nursing is related to a reconnecting, a remembering of its values, traditions and beliefs during a modern century dominated by technology, cure and economic-bureaucratic metaphors which have distorted and silenced nursing's values and practice.*

Given the realities of nursing in the 21st Century, this challenge is more real than ever. Revisiting the BNDU Model of Nursing in contemporary 21st Century nursing and healthcare is an important thing to do, as we increasingly slide into a world of rationalism, pragmatism and genericism! But what we do know more than anything else is that human connection matters and the formation of meaningful connection is core to our being and the foundation upon which excellence in nursing is established.

In recognising the need for an ecological approach to changing systems, Sharmer (2018) proposed 'Theory U' as an awareness-based methodology for changing systems, emphasising the importance of being attentive to our internal world so we can engage wholeheartedly with the external world. The theory is informed by transformative principles of 'being before doing'. Theory U contends that to act effectively we need to know the source/drivers from which we operate when we act, communicate, interpret or think. It is easy to see what we do (results) and how we do it (process), but we are often not aware of the inner drivers for our 'doing' (our practice). These inner drivers can be understood in many ways – values, beliefs, energies, reflectivity, cognition and socialisation to name but a few. Scharmer challenges us to engage in the 'big work' of self-transformation, where we move from a fixed and immutable understanding of practice (i.e. successfully and effectively completing the tasks and interventions of nursing) to one in which we see our practice as the source for maximising individual potential of becoming and evolving into a greater being, i.e. the nurse as a facilitator of human flourishing. In this mode, being and doing are interconnected and guided towards the newly clarified purpose of facilitating flourishing of all persons. With its core question of 'who is this person', the BNDU Model of Nursing acts as an important vehicle for transforming practice from being immutable to person-centred.

The values and principles of the BNDU Model of Nursing are synergistic with principles of person-centredness and the underpinning values of personhood of the Person-centred Practice Framework (PCPF) of McCance and McCormack (2021). We define person-centredness as:

> *an approach to practice established through the formation and fostering of healthful relationships between all care providers, service users and others significant to them in their lives. It is underpinned by values of respect for persons (personhood), individual right to self-determination, mutual respect and understanding. It is enabled by cultures of empowerment that foster continuous approaches to practice development.*

Person-centred practice requires us to connect with our inner-selves as human beings with feelings, emotions, thoughts and desires that guide us as persons. It is the sum of these feelings, emotions, values and desires that guide us towards 'that which really matters' and a connection with our unique humanness as persons – our embodied knowing. The concept of personhood is core to all our being. It is what distinguishes humans from other species. Personhood in its simplest form means being able to reflect on my being in the world – being with my values (what I stand for), being in time (why I respond like I do), being in place (where I am most at ease), being in the social world (how the context influences my behaviour) and being in relation (people I am most authentic with) (Dewing & McCormack 2015). Reflexively understanding my being in the world helps me to know myself as a person and in the context of nursing practice, helps me understand how I can provide person-centred care. Reflective models like the BNDU Model of Nursing bring personhood to life in everyday practice and enable it to be the holistic vehicle for the practice of person-centred nursing.

However, I am also conscious of the burden of responsibility that this places on nurses. Whilst thoughtless practice can never be condoned (such as the personal experience outlined by Chris in Chapter 15) we also know that context matters! Fundamentally, nurses want patients, colleagues and organisations to respect their personhood! As registered nurses providing care, if we are to do so from a person-centred perspective, then we need to work in workplaces and organisations where our personhood is equally valued to that of the patient. To suggest otherwise is to devalue the humanity of registered nurses and compromise their personhood. The importance of person-centred care can never be under-estimated, and we should never take for granted its focus in providing holistic nursing practice. There is ample evidence demonstrating the importance of the existence of a person-centred culture if we are to espouse person-centred care for patients. The person-centred practice framework of McCance and McCormack (2021) has been globally accepted as one theoretical framework that sets out the criteria and qualities that need to be in place for person-centred care to exist and is consistent with the BNDU Model conceptual map set out by Chris in Chapter 15 (page 187). In this framework we articulate the strategic and policy contextual characteristics that governments and other agencies need to put in place to enable organisations to realise a person-centred culture. The framework also highlights the qualities of practitioners that are necessary to be in place to practice person-centredness. However, the framework is also clear that no matter how well developed these qualities, if the practice context is not conducive to this way of practicing, then person-centred care cannot be sustained. We also identify the person-centred processes that healthcare workers need to engage in (irrespective of context or specialty) to facilitate patients experiencing person-centredness and have their personhood respected and nurtured. In the busy, unrelenting, demanding and complex world of everyday practice these demands may seem like idealism, but we know that striving for these ways of being, doing and becoming are core to our personhood and make the difference between us as registered nurses 'doing practice' and being 'engaged with practice'. We also know that the outcome from the implementation of these organisational and practice constructs is that of a 'Healthful Culture' - one in which decision-making is shared, staff relationships are collaborative, leadership is facilitative, innovative practices are supported and it is the ultimate outcome for teams working to develop a workplace that is person-centred. Ultimately a healthful culture leads to the flourishing of all persons.

The BNDU Model of Nursing is being re-published at a critical juncture in the evolution of nursing. This is a time for all nursing leaders to engage in meaningful dialogue about 'what matters' in nursing. Whilst ensuring we achieve the best outcomes for patients, families and communities, we also need to be assertive about the nursing ontological and epistemological foundations upon which such outcomes are achieved. Adopting a holistic and person-centred focus enables us to consider the well-being of all persons and ensure that we are proactively developing workplace cultures that are respectful of all persons and have a central goal of therapeutic effectiveness. Adopting the BNDU model's deeply reflective approach to our practice could be a vehicle for significant transformation in nursing. As Pema Chödrön (2020: 9) asserts:

"When things are shaky and nothing is working, we might realize that we are on the verge of something. We might realize that this is a very vulnerable and tender place, and that tenderness can go either way. We can shut down and feel resentful or we can touch in on that throbbing quality."

REFERENCES

Chödrön, P (2020) When Things Fall Apart: Heart Advice for Difficult Times. Colorado: Shambhala.

Dewing J and McCormack B (2015) A critique of the concept of engagement and its application in person-centred practice. International Practice Development Journal http://www.fons.org/library/journal/volume5-person-centredness-suppl/article6

McCance, T. and McCormack, B. (2021) The Person-centred Practice Framework, in McCormack B, McCance T, Martin S, McMillan A, Bulley C (2021) Fundamentals of Person-centred Healthcare Practice Wiley, Oxford. PP: 23-32 https://www.perlego.com/book/2068078/fundamentals-of-personcentred-healthcare-practice-pdf?utm_source=google&utm_medium=cpc&gclid=Cj0KCQjwtrSLBhCLARIsACh6Rmj9sarf1IjwEHCseXMsPLGeUTTQlJWYL6mfQEQgwO3ln-LkUU9Gb0A8aAgT1EALw_wcB

Scharmer, C.O. (2018) The Essentials of Theory U: Core Principles and Applications. Oakland CA: Berrett-Koehler Publishers.

Preface

Last year I was invited to become an honorary scholar of the Global Academy of Holistic Nursing in recognition of my work developing holistic practice. At the 2022 online induction ceremony I was invited to give the end-note address. I chose to tell the Burford story. I realised it remains relevant, perhaps even more so, to inform and influence healthcare practice.

The Burford NDU Model: Caring in Practice was published by Blackwell Science in 1994. The model is grounded in Burford practitioners' collective holistic vision and ensuing systems to enable the vision to be realised in everyday practice. This revised edition is not a prescription of how to *do* holistic practice. It is an invitation for readers to dialogue with the text to inform your practice, whether you are a practitioner, teacher or organizer, towards realising holistic practice as a lived reality.

The term 'holistic practice' was used throughout the original text. Since then I preferred the term *person-centred practice* as it seemed to be more direct for practitioners to understand. Holism may seem too abstract, especially within a British nursing culture focused more on what I do rather than what I believe. But I return to the word *holism*. Being person-centred is integral to being holistic. A word holds meaning and I sense holism is a powerful word. It is about perceiving the bigger picture.

Scanning Amazon there are numerous references to person-centred practice published in the UK over the past few years that indicate the significance of this approach to current healthcare practice, not least by McCormack (2021), McCormack and McCance (2016). The emergence of the International Community of Practice spanning different countries is committed to developing person-centred practice.[1] However, there is considerably less reference to holistic practice in the UK, although commonly referenced in the USA. Hence the distinction between the two concepts appears to be largely cultural.

Without doubt, a holistic vision is compelling. Most nursing and other health care practitioners aspire to realising it. Why would anyone choose nursing as a profession if they didn't want to practice holistic care? However, we might commence nurse training motivated with a notion of caring, yet through training and organizational conditioning, this caring can fade in light of reality. Thus both the way nurses are trained and organizational practices need to shift to meaningfully and practically cultivate holistic practice. Although this is obvious, in reality it is challenging due to deeply entrenched tradition. The basic question remains as valid today as in 1994 – that if we value and aspire to holistic practice, how can it be *truly* realised within everyday practice? I italicise *truly* because no doubt many practitioners across health care professions believe their practice is holistic. Of course this question challenges that practitioners have a sense of what holistic practice looks like and experienced.

ROOTS

Burford Community hospital was nestled in the rural Cotswold Hills of Oxfordshire. It became well known as a centre of innovative practice from 1983 through the work of Alan Pearson (1983) who established its status as a nursing development unit. Pearson (1988) had researched the development of nursing beds with nursing as a primary therapy based on the vision of the Loeb Center in New York (Hall 1964). He introduced primary nursing at Burford that shifted the culture of the hospital from its previous task approach to practice. Pearson departed in 1986 to establish a companion nursing development unit at the Radcliffe Infirmary in Oxford. Investment in nursing development in Oxford during this time was a significant factor fuelled by wider developments in nursing with the advent of nursing models, nursing diagnosis, the nursing process and primary nursing. These ideas all focused on the development of nursing as a profession.

Arriving at Burford in 1989, I commenced a process of reflection on the nature and delivery of clinical practice at Burford. The recognition of being a nursing development unit with its achievement through Pearson's work created the expectation that the Burford NDU would pursue an active developmental role.

POSING THE QUESTION

Consider - 'What do you, the reader, aspire to achieve when you pull on your uniform?' 'What are your beliefs about the nature of your practice?' 'Are your beliefs realised in everyday practice?' 'What needs to change to realise your beliefs?'

Clearly the rhetoric of holistic practice is a powerful influence. Yet aspiration needs articulating. Then it needs realising.

There is much media reports that healthcare and nursing practice is far from satisfactory. Just last week, Panorama[2] revealed their undercover exposure of care at Edenfield hospital in the UK. It was shocking. How can nurses practice like that? How does the practice environment become so toxic? The fact is that practice easily becomes routine where people, both staff and patients, are reduced to objects. Caring becomes non-caring, adding to suffering for both patients and practitioners. Morale plummets. Sickness rates rise. Practitioners go through the motions.

I know this from my own experience and my retort that 'people are not numbers to crunch' (Johns and Rose 2022) where we had become objects in an illness fixing machine and where nurses were blind. On sharing this narrative as a performance, a member of the audience poignantly noted (p. 141):

> *I'm a nurse matron of acute medicine. What you portray is most uncomfortable. It has really made me think. What makes nurses blind in my view, is the way care has become so routinised and so unreflective because of the need to get through the work and poor leadership. It has become a pervasive and perverted culture. Also our systems are inadequate if they don't guide the nurse to consider how the person is feeling like 'nurse fantastic' in the performance. Not that a nurse should need guiding. It should be a built in as a natural way to approach the person. I feel so very sorry for Otter and yourself for experiencing that.*

Clearly there is a massive problem within organizations to allow this 'perverse and pervasive' practice to exist and persist. Every person who requires health care deserves holistic practice. There are no excuses even when practice is under pressure. Yet I sense that nothing much has changed over the past thirty years. Many nurses are not blind although they may turn a blind eye. I meet many nurses who want to give holistic care and yet they practice in situations that constrain this. As Jonathan, an advanced nurse practitioner admitting me for an appendicectomy recently responded after I had informed him that he was the first nurse to introduce himself (three previous nurses had failed to this) "I know, it's not good enough, all the good ones leave." It's as if nurses fit-in to whatever system exists, without any power to shift this. Without doubt, health care practice has become increasingly corporate with emphasis on outcomes or targets with finite resources and staff shortages that makes practice reactive rather than proactive, task driven rather than creative, managerially driven rather than leadership, risk adverse rather than therapeutic; factors all contributing to caring being a lottery rather than committed intent.

It requires organizations to wake up to the challenge and invest in people towards realising holistic practice, to realise their own vision statements that espouse holistic or person-centred practice. It requires a holistic type of leadership to work with practitioners through creating a vision of holistic practice and to develop systems to facilitate its realization. This leadership should be at every level of the organization to create a dynamic learning organization.

It requires teachers to re-vision the curriculum around reflection and holistic values to prepare practitioners to become holistic practitioners with close links to clinical practice working with organisations to ensure students learn in holistic environments.

HOLISTIC KNOWING

Eduardo Chillida (2019:48) jotted:

> *The artist (and we can say the practitioner is an artist) knows what he's doing, but for it to be worthwhile, he must take the leap and do what he doesn't know how to do. In that moment, he is beyond knowledge.*

So every day make the leap with the intention to be holistic. Your performance as a practitioner is art in motion. Holism is a way of being in the world that is often ineffable, beyond words, informed by knowledge yet transcending knowledge – knowing something directly through experiencing it [knowing how] more than knowing something indirectly through information [knowing that]. Knowing something through experience can be made more explicit through reflection whereby the practitioner's knowing becomes a self-inquiry to gain insight to inform future practice. Such knowing is largely intuitive within the moment. We may have ideas about what holistic practice is but that's not the same as living it. Obviously ideas inform but we can only know something through doing it. Hence the significance of reflection as feedback – "How do I know if I am realising holistic practice?' You can read books about it, you might gain some ideas about it but they won't tell you what it is like to be a holistic practitioner.

As Yoko Beck notes (1989:123)

> *Suppose we want to realise how a marathon runner feels; if we run two blocks, or two miles or five miles, we will know something about running those distances, but we won't know anything about running a marathon. We can recite theories about marathons; we can describe tables about the physiology of marathon runners; we can pile up endless information about marathon-running; but that doesn't mean we know what it is. We can only know when we are the one doing it. We only know our lives when we experience them directly, instead of dreaming about how they might be if we did this, or had that. This we can call running in place, being present to we are, right here and right now.*

THE BURFORD NDU MODEL: AN OVERVIEW

The core of the Burford NDU model is a collective holistic vision of practice reflecting the beliefs of Burford practitioners to give meaning and direction to their practice. Practitioners are guided to live the vision through five systems set within the dynamic learning culture and holistic leadership.

However, practice is not rationale but steeped deeply in issues of power, tradition and embodiment that must be understood and shifted as necessary to accommodate holistic practice (Fay 1987). As the book unfolds the reader will grasp the necessary shift in culture to effectively accommodate holistic practice.

However, the Burford NDU model is simply a structure. It can be adapted to 'fit' other practice settings who aspire to holistic practice. Some practice settings may simply 'take it of the shelf' and apply in a functional way as they might any other idea although the model's impact on enabling holistic practice may be limited.

STRUCTURE OF THE BOOK

The whole book is a reflective and holistic text. It explores the pattern of systems within the whole, patterns that are essentially tentative and moveable, always reflected on and developed to support holistic practice.

Jean Watson writes one foreword to this new edition just as she wrote the original preface bridging the time span between texts. Brendan McCormack writes a second foreword alongside his original engagement with the Buford NDU model again spanning time between texts. Both are world leaders and activists in developing holistic practice globally. Their words are inspirational and set the scene for the book's unfolding.

In Chapter 1, I set out a holistic vision of practice and how this was constructed at Burford hospital to become the foundation of the Burford NDU holistic model for practice. I argue that a vision needs to be valid, addressing the nature of caring, the internal environment of practice and its social viability. I also argue that a vision needs to be 'collective', owned by practitioners.

In Chapter 2, I set out the Burford NDU model evolving from Burford hospital's vision for practice as the structure to enable practitioners to realise their holistic vision as a lived reality. The model comprises five systems set within a culture of a dynamic learning culture driven by 'holistic' leadership reflecting a synchronicity between process (organising holistic practice) and outcome (realising holistic practice). Yet realising holistic practice is not a rational process. It requires a significant culture shift moving from a prevailing dominant task focused functional culture to delivering clinical practice. As such, the holistic leader is a dynamic change agent. As such, the whole book is a template for guiding practitioners and organizations through change. It is reflective rather than prescriptive, opening possibilities.

In Chapters 3–7, I set out the five systems designed to enable the Burford hospital vision to be realised in everyday practice.

Chapter 3 sets out the pattern appreciation or assessment strategy to tune practitioners into the holistic vision and guide practitioners to gather necessary information to nurse the person as an ongoing dynamic process throughout the person's journey in hospital and beyond. It is this aspect of the Burford model that most likely will attract potential users due to its profound simplicity and meaningful practicality.

Chapter 4 sets out a system for reflexive communication. Reflexivity is looking back in the present moment whilst anticipating moving forward. Dialogue is the mode of communication both verbal and written as an unfolding narrative that tells the story of working with the person.

In Chapter 5, I advocate primary nursing as the most appropriate system to deliver holistic practice because it best facilitates the relationship between the practitioner and the person in contrast with other approaches. However, primary nursing needs to be supported by the therapeutic team. However, this is not without its challenges, notably the emergence of 'ownership' whereby associate nurses can feel 'pushed out' and 'unacknowledged' for their contribution, and the 'harmonious team' with its consequence of practitioners not being available to each other, dealing effectively with situations of conflict, and giving and receiving feedback.

Chapter 6 sets out guided reflection as the system to enable practitioners to realise the Burford NDU model supported by three scenarios recorded from guided reflection sessions. It makes absolute sense that a practice discipline such as nursing ground learning in its practice. This account of guided reflection is brief. The reader is referred to my book *Becoming a Reflective Practitioner* (Johns 2022) for an in-depth exploration of learning through reflection from both educational and clinical settings.

Chapter 7 sets out a system for living and ensuring quality whereby quality of care is everyone's business moment by moment facilitated by everyday talk both formal and informal, guided reflection, standards of care and clinical audit. In fact every aspect of practice is concerned with clinical effectiveness and practitioner performance.

Chapters 8–10 are written by Buford practitioners reflecting on working with the Burford model. These chapters are reproduced from the 1994 version accompanied by new footnotes to draw out significance. They offer critical insight into living the Burford NDU model to enable readers to contextually sense the nature of holistic practice and what it means to be a holistic practitioner alongside the practicality of the Burford NDU model to facilitate it. As the reader will appreciate, it is not all plain sailing. The accounts reveal that it can be difficult and painful at times reflecting how old ways of practice are difficult to shift. It is the commitment to holistic practice that enables these practitioners to prevail in hard times – because the joy in practicing holistically far outweighs any difficulty.

Chapters 11–13 are written by practitioners from other practice settings who critically reflect on implementing the Burford NDU model, offering their own insights and adaptations to suit their local practice from different practice settings. One setting is a comparable Community hospital to Burford. Another setting is an acute medical ward within a large general hospital. The third setting is a district nursing practice.

As with Chapters 8–10 I have written footnotes to draw out significance.

Chapter 14 is my reflection on my practice as a holistic therapist in a hospice setting that had implemented the Burford NDU model although without a collective vision. I draw out significant aspects of what it means to be a holistic practitioner working autonomously yet within the multi-disciplinary team. The narrative conveys that the individual practitioner can approach their practice with holistic intent even for brief moments and where holistic beliefs are not collective. However, the narrative also suggests the struggle such individuals face where holistic beliefs are not collective.

In Chapter 15, I coin the mantra 'holistic practice matters'. It explores the consequences of holistic practice from political, organizational and educational perspectives returning to the question – can holistic practice ever be a reality in everyday health care practice or will it always be a compelling pipe dream of the way practice ought to be but ultimately fall upon stony ground? In drawing together the threads of the book I set out a conceptual map and argue that the truth of realising holistic practice lies essentially with practitioner accounts. Finally the chapter is an invitation to dialogue.

So this book, a 30th anniversary review and development of the Burford NDU holistic model, asserts itself as a challenge to all practitioners, organizations and universities to wake up and heed the call towards enabling practitioners to become holistic practitioners and in doing so, to unleash their therapeutic potential for the benefit of people everywhere and, in doing so, to realise their professional destiny.

In the words of Martin Luther King, Jr.:

This is no time for apathy or complacency. This is a time for vigorous and positive action.[3]

I have tended to use the term 'practitioners' suggesting that holistic practice is not just the concern of nurses but for all healthcare disciplines. Obviously my background is as a nurse and it is nurses that set the environmental tone of practice settings.

I am mindful of the British-centric nature of the text. International readers will be aware of that to reflect on how the text can inform their own cultural practices.

Readers will note that many references are dated to the era of the original text. This gives a flavour of the background to the model's development and its relevance for today's nursing and health care practice. Readers inspired to explore and implement holistic practice can search a more recent literature. A notable example is the text by McCormack et al (2021). The inside flap states 'Fundamentals of Person-Centred Healthcare Practice presents evidence-based perspectives on a broad range of approaches to person-centred practice in healthcare'.

NOTES

1 The International Community of Practice for Person-centred Practice (PcP-ICoP) is an international community of collaborating organisations committed to improving the understanding of person-centredness and its advancement in clinical practice, research, education/learning, facilitation, management, policy and strategy.

McCormack B and Dewing J (2019) International Community of Practice for Person-centred Practice: position statement on person-centredness in health and social care3. International Practice Development Journal 9.1.3. (https://doi.org/10.19043/ipdj.91.003)

2 BBC Panorama Undercover Hospital: Patients at Risk – Thursday 29th September 2022. [https://www.bbc.news.com]

There have been many exposures of poor healthcare. People often complain about care. The report 'A Review of the NHS Hospitals Complaints System; Putting Patients Back in the Picture' [October 2013] states: 'One of the most shocking failures in NHS care was documented on 6th February 2013 when Robert Francis QC published his Public Inquiry into Mid Staffordshire NHS Foundation Trust. He found a story of appalling and unnecessary suffering of hundreds of people.

To quote

'They were failed by a system which ignored the warning signs and put corporate self-interest and cost control ahead of patients and their safety. A health service that does not listen to complaints is unlikely to reflect its patients' needs. One that does will be more likely to detect the early warning signs that something requires correction, to address such issues and to protect others from harmful treatment. A complaints system that does not respond flexibly, promptly and effectively to the justifiable concerns of complainants not only allows unacceptable practice to persist, it aggravates the grievance and suffering of the patient and those associated with the complaint, and undermines the public's trust in the service'.

This review was co-chaired by Ann Clwyd MP. In a radio interview on BBC Radio 4's World at One in December 2012, she described the way in which her husband, Owen Roberts, had died in the University Hospital of Wales. Ann Clwyd spoke of the "coldness, resentment, indifference and contempt" of some of the nurses who were supposed to be caring for him. She broke down in tears as she recalled his last hours, shivering under flimsy sheets, with an ill-fitting oxygen mask cutting into his face, wedged up against the bars of the hospital bed. She said her husband, a former head of News and Current Affairs for BBC Wales, died "like a battery hen."

Following this programme and others she received letters and emails from hundreds of people who were appalled at such a lapse in standards of basic decency and compassion. Many included accounts of other shocking examples of poor care and of the difficulty people encountered when trying to complain. The report noted that more than 2500 testimonials were received from patients, their relatives, friends or carers. The majority describe problems with the quality of treatment or care in NHS hospitals. Key points raised:

- Lack of information – patients said they felt uninformed about their care and treatment.
- Compassion – patients said they felt they had not been treated with the compassion they deserve.
- Dignity and care – patients said they felt neglected and not listened to.
- Staff attitudes – patients said they felt no one was in charge on the ward and the staff were too busy to care for them.
- Resources – patients said there was a lack of basic supplies like extra blankets and pillows.

3 King M L Jr. (1958) Stride towards freedom. Harper & Row Publishers, London.

REFERENCES

Beck C J (1989) *Everyday Zen*. Thorsons, London.

Chillida E (2019) *Writings*. La Frabrica Madrid/ Hauser and Wirth Publishers.

Hall L (1964) Nursing- what is it? *The Canadian Nurse*, 60(2) 250-4.

Johns C and Rose O (2022) 'People are not numbers to crunch': a performance narrative and storyboard. In *Becoming a reflective practitioner (sixth edition)* (Ed. C Johns) Wilery Blackwell, Oxford, p133–142.

McCormack B and McCance T (2016) *Person-Centred Practice in Nursing and Health Care: Theory and Practice*. Wiley-Blackwell, Oxford.

McCormack B, McCance T, Bulley C, Brown D, McMillan A and Martin S (Eds.) (2021) *Fundamentals of Person-Centred Healthcare Practice: A Guide for Healthcare Students*. Wiley Blackwell, Oxford.

Pearson A (1983) *The clinical nursing unit*. Heinemann Medical Books, London.

Pearson A (1988) *Primary nursing in the Burford and Oxford Nursing Development Units*. Croom Helm, Sydney.

Acknowledgments

I am deeply indebted to Jean Watson and Brendan McCormack for their forewords in supporting this book. Jean wrote the foreword for the original book in 1994 and Brendan contributed a chapter with his colleagues on implementing the Burford NDU model within OXCOMM community hospital.

To Jan Dewing

One of the contributors to the first edition of the BNDU Model of Nursing text was Professor Jan Dewing. Jan died in August 2022 aged 61. Prior to her untimely death, Jan was the Sue Pembrey Chair in Nursing and Director of the Centre for Person-centred Practice Research https://www.cpcpr.org/ at Queen Margaret University, Edinburgh, where she was also Head of the University's Graduate Research School. She was a leading scholar in person-centred practice, with a particular focus on people living with dementia. Jan worked with health and social care teams nationally and internationally to ensure care was delivered in a way that respected who the person was. When the first edition of the BNDU Model of Nursing was published, Jan was a lecturer/practitioner with young people living with disabilities and she worked closely with Chris Johns in Clinical Supervision and supported reflective practice. Later, Jan went on to replace Chris as the Nurse Manager at Burford Nursing Development Unit and built on the work that Chris had started. Her vision and passion for this work resulted in it being spread across all community hospitals in Oxfordshire. It was my privilege to work closely with her in doing this and to continue to work with her as a close friend and colleague until her death. Jan was a living example of the BNDU model in action and she has influenced so many people in these ways of working around the world and her legacy will live on for a very long time yet!

To Helen Erikson, Executive director of the Global Academy of Holistic Nursing, who drew me into the Academy and prompted my writing this book.

To all those at Wiley Blackwell who made this book possible, notably. Executive Editor, Tom Marriott, Managing Editor, Bhavya Bhoopathi and Content Operation Specialist, Krithika Shivakumar and Wiley's creative and production teams.

Finally to Otter, my partner, supporter and critic, always challenging ideas for their reality.

Holistic or Person-centred Vision for Practice

CHAPTER 1

Christopher Johns

The foundation of the Burford NDU model is a vision or philosophy for practice. In the first edition of this book I adopted the term 'a philosophy for practice'. I prefer 'vision' because it suggests being able to see the way ahead, that practitioners are not blind to their practice but have their eyes and minds wide open to pay attention and be curious about their practice.

Holding a vision of practice gives meaning and purpose to everyday practice. It makes it more likely that practitioners collectively pull together in the same direction leading to more consistent and congruent practice. As a written statement, it is a constant reminder to practitioners of what they seek to realise in their everyday practice. Constructing a vision wakes practitioners up! It is confrontational. It makes them think and reflect.

Ask yourself:

- 'What are your beliefs and values about your practice?'
- 'Are these beliefs and values important for you to realise?'
- 'Do you actually realise these beliefs in your everyday practice?'
- 'What needs to change to realise your beliefs as a lived reality?'

COMMENCING AT THE BEGINNING

Prior to my arrival at Burford hospital, the hospital's vision of practice was based on Lydia Hall's philosophy of the Loeb Centre in New York (Hall 1964, Alfano 1971). Hall's work was a vision of nursing as the primary therapy alongside a complementary role to medicine. In 1982, when Pearson (1983) introduced this philosophy to Burford, it made sense in terms of his intent to establish nursing beds. Yet, three years after Pearson's departure, when I asked practitioners to tell me about the hospital's philosophy the Loeb vision had faded. Practitioners who remained from that era vaguely remembered bits of it. It was no longer alive. It did not reflect current practice and hence, was no longer relevant. As one practitioner responded 'It was imported by the hospital manager and had little relevance to the other staff. It was his vision'.

I surmised that an imported philosophy imposes a reality on practitioners that denies the expression of their own beliefs or indeed, may contradict them. As such, they could only comply with it or passively ignore it.

Holistic Practice in Healthcare: The Burford NDU Person-centred Model, Second Edition. Edited by Christopher Johns.

My view is that the hospital's vision should collectively reflect the beliefs and values of its practitioners or put another way be 'tailor made' to fit the practice setting.

The value in doing that is reflected in Senge's words (1990:206/8)

> *When people truly share a vision they are connected, bound together by a common aspiration. Visions are exhilarating... they create the 'spark', the excitement that lifts an organization out of the mundane.*

The *'spark'* energises practitioners. It stirs them from complacency. It fires commitment; that the vision matters. Without commitment, practitioners simply wouldn't bother, taking the path of least resistance for a quiet life.

Commitment is achieved by being part of the vision, of having contributed to it and knowing it reflects one's own beliefs. When all involved share a collective vision then the energy created is more than the sum of the individuals. Practitioners gain a real sense of belonging to a team dedicated to realising the vision as a lived reality. A positive and creative buzz about the place! Practice becomes exciting and paradoxically easier simply because practitioners are liberated to practice their beliefs.

The written vision offers a public statement to which others – patients, families, the local community, the wider society and all health care disciplines can relate to. It sets up the basis for dialogue, expectation and collaboration. It becomes the foundation stone for all clinical practice and practice development.

CONSTRUCTING THE HOLISTIC VISION

For clarity, constructing the vision at Burford hospital can be viewed as moving through six steps:

Step 1

The first step is to generate a 'felt need[1]' for a new vision that reflects practitioners' beliefs about practice at Burford. I instigated conversations with staff to critically reflect on the meaning of their practice – 'What are your beliefs about nursing at Burford?' As Senge (1990:211) notes 'If people don't have their own vision, all they can do is sign up for someone else's. The result is compliance, never commitment.' Having a personal vision is significant in contributing to a wider collaborative vision.

A typical practitioner response was 'to care for the patient?' In response I inquire 'tell me about this caring?' Usually, the response was in terms of what the practitioner 'did', rather than their beliefs. So I would push the conversation towards beliefs. It was like unlocking a door to the mind, to get practitioners to really think about their practice, perhaps for the first time.

From these conversations I appreciated that articulating their beliefs was not easy for some practitioners. I recognised this difficulty of articulation was that practitioners' perceptions of nursing have been dominated by a functional rather than beliefs conception. This was not surprising given the prevailing 'task' culture of nursing at Burford – 'this is what we always do' reflecting how practice was unreflective and largely taken for granted.

One reason why nursing is functional is that it has traditionally been organised through prescribed tasks beneath the shadow of a dominant culture of the medical model and transactional management culture of 'getting through the work'.

Within this culture, nurses have suppressed their own beliefs as relatively unimportant. This parallels suspension of the rights of people expected to respond as good patients to investigation and treatment responses. Nursing's primary role has been to support this endeavour – hence the idea of the doctor's handmaiden. Caring is then a sub-culture, furtively taking place alongside the real work of supporting the medical agenda. Nurses like patients are expected to be submissive. As such, nursing as 'caring' has not been really valued by the organisation or by nurses themselves.

Step 2

To engage all staff in expressing their beliefs about Burford practice I posted two sheets of flipchart paper on the wall and invited all staff to contribute vision statements no matter their role. To get people started I added two of my own:

- 'I believe we should be of service to our patients and to one another.'
- 'I believe in creating and sustaining a learning community where we grow individually and together to become most responsible and effective.'

Step 3

Over the following weeks practitioners slowly added their beliefs. The flipchart created its own curiosity and interest as more statements of beliefs were added.

Step 4

After two months, I convened two community meetings to explore the beliefs, ensuring that no belief was dismissed. The beliefs all pointed towards holistic practice in terms of caring for the person. I pointed out that a need for reciprocity between caring for persons and for ourselves – 'How can others be cared for if those caring are not likewise cared for?' I felt this should be explicit within the vision. However, whilst I had such ideas, I was careful not to impose them like a dictator. I felt I also needed to paint the bigger picture of placing 'caring' within an ideological, historical, cultural, societal and organisational context of health care as visions do not exist in a vacuum but are subject to such influences. For example, 'what are the expectations of the local community of its community hospital?'

From an ideological and societal perspective, health care had shifted towards a patient experience perspective, shifting the relationship between health care practitioner and the patient. Hence being person-centred rode this perspective. It gave credibility to a shift in the hospital vision. In other words, I needed to paint this bigger picture in which to frame our collective beliefs towards constructing our collaborative vision. It needed to be possible to realise rather than fanciful or idealistic.

Step 5

I constructed a composite of the stated beliefs around the focus of holistic practice. I gave each person a copy for comment, to amend as necessary and reach consensus at a subsequent community meeting.

Step 6

The first draft was discussed and criticised for being too jardonistic, especially as we were going to share this vision with the general public as a statement of what to expect from the hospital. This was revised and agreed. The vision was realised (Figure 1.1).

The process of writing the vision took four months. It opened a learning space for all practitioners to voice their views and reflect on their collective practice. It enabled practitioners to find voice and become active creators of their own practice and take responsibility for realising *their* vision as a lived reality in their everyday practice. Most of all this collective work created a community of learning. No longer was practice taken for granted. Practitioners now had a greater sense of purpose. There was a buzz about the place. Having written their vision I could then point towards holistic literature (collected in the hospital library) to deepen their interest and contrast with our vision.

We believe our care is holistic, grounded in the core therapeutic of easing suffering and enabling the growth of the other through his/ her health-illness experience whether toward recovery or death. The practitioner is mindful of being of service and being available to work with the person and the person's family in relationship, whereby the person's life pattern and health needs are appreciated and effectively responded to on the basis of mutual understanding.

Caring is seamless across health care settings and responds to and promotes both the local community's and society's expectations of effective service. In this respect, we accept a responsibility to develop a culture of reflective leadership and the learning organisation that continually strives to anticipate and develop practice to ensure its efficacy and quality. By appropriate monitoring and sharing, we contribute to the development of the societal value of nursing and health care generally.

Our caring is enhanced when we work in dialogical relationship with our [multi] professional colleagues on the basis of mutual respect and shared values within our respective roles. This means being free to share our feelings openly but appropriately, acknowledging that as persons, we can be stressed and have differences of opinion at times. This is the basis of the therapeutic team that is essential to reciprocate and support our caring to patients.

[March 2003, amended 2012, 2015]

FIGURE 1.1 Burford vision for clinical practice [4th edition]

VALID VISION

Yet what should a vision state to be valid? I discerned that a vision for practice needed to address three 'cornerstones' [Figure 1.2].

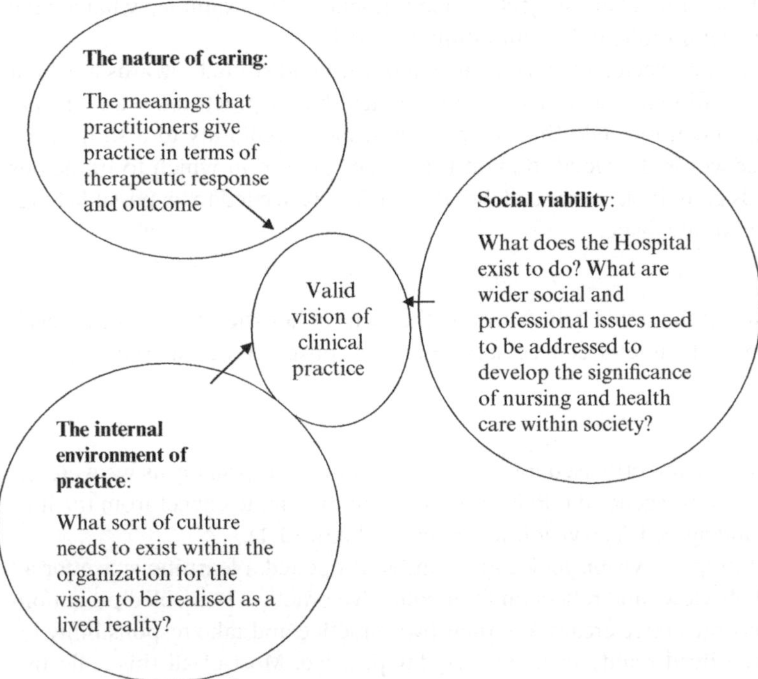
The nature of caring:
The meanings that practitioners give practice in terms of therapeutic response and outcome
Valid vision of clinical practice
Social viability:
What does the Hospital exist to do? What are wider social and professional issues need to be addressed to develop the significance of nursing and health care within society?
The internal environment of practice:
What sort of culture needs to exist within the organization for the vision to be realised as a lived reality?

FIGURE 1.2 Cornerstones of a valid vision.

THE NATURE OF CARING

Constructing a vision challenges practitioners to think about their beliefs about the nature of their clinical practice. It seems axiomatic that *caring* is the foundational ontological substance of nursing and underpins nursing's epistemology (Watson 1990). As Carper (1978:12) informs –

> *Caring, as a professional and personal value, is of central importance in providing a normative standard which governs our action and out attitudes to those for whom we care.*

I would challenge any practitioner to doubt the truth of these words. Yet what is caring? The word 'caring' resonates through the Burford vision. It explicitly espouses a *holistic* vision of caring practice. It acknowledges that people suffer. Suffering can be viewed as a disruption of the whole person that manifests on the physical, emotional, psychological and spiritual planes.

HOLISM

Holism is seeing and responding to the person as a 'whole' person, whereby the whole is greater than the sum of its parts. Holistic practice is actualised through the relationship between the practitioner(s) and person(s) requiring help to meet their health-illness needs and, in doing so, ease suffering and grow through the experience. This relationship is 'working with' the person based on negotiating the person's needs (as able) through dialogue and in collaboration with other health professionals.

Jean Watson (1988:49[2]) expands the idea of holism –

> *The goal of nursing proposed is to help persons gain a higher degree of harmony within the mind, body and soul which generates self-knowledge, self-reverence, self-healing and self-care processes while allowing increasing diversity. This goal is pursued through the human-human caring process and caring transactions that respond to the subjective inner world of the person in such a way that the nurse helps individuals find meaning in their existence, disharmony, suffering, and turmoil and promotes self-control, choice, and self-determination with the health-illness decisions.*

Compared with the Burford vision statement, Watson's words are very different and yet essentially say the same thing. In particular the notion of the *human-human encounter* essential in working with the person on the basis of mutual understanding. Watson's words challenge the reader to think differently about the 'nature of nursing', opening the mind to possibility and challenging previous ways of perceiving practice.

McCormack et al. (2021) identify the core values of person-centred practice that again are largely reflected in the Burford vision. These core values are; respect for personhood, being authentic, sharing autonomy, showing respect for and active engagement with the person's individual abilities, preferences, lifestyles and goals, demonstrating mutual respect and understanding, and committed to healthfulness as process and outcome

What Watson and McCormack et al. write about holism or person-centred practice are powerful influences on practitioners' perception of nursing, although I strongly urge practitioners to first explore their own views rather than be caught up by the words of others.

THE SCOPE OF HOLISTIC INTERVENTIONS

Neuman's (1980) typology of nursing interventions enables practitioners to perceive the scope of interventions from a holistic perspective:

Primary– aimed to appreciate and strengthen the resistance of the person to factors that cause suffering and illness.
Secondary– aimed to respond most effectively to the symptoms of suffering and illness
Tertiary– aimed to enable the person learn and grow through their health-illness experience to realise a more satisfactory life pattern.

RESPECTING AUTONOMY AND ETHICAL DECISION-MAKING

Holistic practice is ethical practice – knowing the right response in terms of acting for the best informed as appropriate by ethical principles. Every situation is unique requiring the practitioner to judge the notion of 'what is the best response' in dialogue with the person. Working with the person respects their autonomy to make decisions about their life (Seedhouse 1988). However, the primacy of person autonomy may create conflict with practitioners who consider that they know what is best for the person. Differences of opinion are bound to occur with both the person and with the person's family. The holistic practitioner surfaces the conflict so it can be seen for what it is diffusing any emotional fall-out as necessary to guide people involved to resolution.

A second principle to appreciate is utilitarianism – the notion of acting for the greatest good with finite resources notably when workload is heavy and demand from persons can feel overwhelming. This can naturally create a tension with the notion of meeting person's needs – reinforcing the significance of working with the person to ensure care is negotiated.

THE HOLISTIC ORGANISATION

Holism also applies to the organisation, not just clinical practice. The holistic organisation is a 'whole' and all staff, resources and systems parts within it. It requires a holistic leadership to see and enable others to see the bigger picture as a background to all activity within it (I explore holistic leadership in Chapter 2).

STARK CONTRAST

In constructing a holistic vision for practice it is necessary to understand the existing state of affairs within the practice unit in order to envisage the necessary shift of culture to realise holistic practice. For many Units, holistic practice is a stark contrast with the prevailing functional approach of the medical model whereby the ill person is reduced to the status of a patient with a set of symptoms that require investigation, diagnosis and subsequent treatment. Little significance is attributed to emotional, psychological, spiritual and social aspects of being ill or causes of illness. The nursing response is primarily to support the medical task and authority. I am sure many readers will remember being told not to sit on the bed and talk to the patient – 'there is work to be done!' The implication being is that talking to patients is not real work. The rise of technology and squeeze on resources has led to a culture whereby caring has been increasingly subordinated to unqualified staff. When the head is locked into the medical sphere and the medical sphere is most valued within organisations, then practitioners will lose sight of the holistic ideal. I know many readers will have experienced this state of affairs when visiting family or friends, or experienced their own heath care.

Yet in a world where the health agenda is dominated by productivity, and a culture of 'more for less', times are hard for caring. Practitioners may switch off their caring self, simply because it is too painful to witness suffering and the failure to ease it.

HOLISTIC CONCEPTS

A number of concepts integral to holistic practice require deeper understanding. These concepts became apparent from an analysis of practitioners' reflections of experiences shared within guided reflection (the focus of Chapter 6) in dialogue with relevant theory as part of my doctoral research (Johns 1998).

- Being available
- Situated meaning
- Working with relationship
- Tuning in or wavelength theory
- Being fully present
- Professional involvement (balancing concern and poise)
- Lifting energy
- Enabling growth
- Journeying

BEING AVAILABLE

Burford's vision states, 'The practitioner is mindful of being available to work with the person.' To be available requires turning one's attention toward the person, being aware of and open to the 'here and now' shared situation, and communicating one's availability. It is saying to the person 'I am here for you when you need me'.

However, to be realistic, the person must also appreciate the pressure on the practitioner to manage a workload and meet the needs of other persons. Through involvement, the person can also care for the practitioner. Care being a mutual process from a holistic perspective yet without any expectation that the person should care for the practitioner.

Table 1.1 The being available template

Attribute	Comment
The extent the practitioner holds holistic intent	The practitioner approaches every clinical situation mindful of being a holistic practitioner. In other words holism shifts from an idea to apply to become a state of being developed through reflection.
The extent the practitioner is fully present to the person	To be *fully present* it is necessary to clear the mind from distraction – what I term 'bringing the mind home'. It acknowledges that the practitioner's mind is often full of stuff that interferes with being fully present.
The extent the practitioner knows the person	The practitioner appreciates the pattern of the person's wholeness and *situation* and the meanings they give to their health-illness experience by *tuning into and flowing with the person's wavelength* throughout the person's shifting health-illness experience.
The extent the practitioner is concerned for the person[4]	*Concern* reflects that the person matters to the practitioner. It is an energy that creates possibility and lifts people (see lifting energy below).
The extent the practitioner is effective in meeting the person's needs	The practitioner's *works with* the person (as able) to effectively meet their needs as a continuous process by: • Appreciating the person's needs (primary, secondary and tertiary) • Responding with appropriate, ethical and skilful action • Evaluating whether the person's needs have been effectively met
The extent the practitioner is poised	Poise is the practitioner's ability to know and manage self so that any distractions, feelings or emotions do not interfere with being available to the person. It is the flip side of concern, whereas concern makes the practitioner vulnerable, so poise manages the vulnerability without diminishing concern enabling professional involvement.
The extent the practitioner can create and sustain an environment where being available is possible	Practice takes place within an environmental setting that impacts on the practitioner being available. The practitioner accepts responsibility for working with colleagues to ensure that all aspects of the practice environment best facilitates being available.

(Adapted from Johns 2022.)[3]

The person is the more vulnerable partner in their relationship with the practitioner. It is the person who requires the practitioner's expertise. As such, the holistic practitioner is mindful of putting the person at ease without any authoritative pressure. The practitioner acts to enable the voice of the person to speak their authentic self by revealing her own authentic self. However, self-disclosure is not an open tap. It is always deliberate and purposeful.

The extent the practitioner can be available is influenced by a number of attributes (Table 1.1). In considering these attributes it is important to keep in mind that they are *aspects of the whole*, rather than be viewed in isolation. They are dynamic parts in constant movement forming a holistic caring pattern.

SITUATED MEANING

The practitioner's perception of the 'whole' person is viewed within the context of the person's particular situation. Benner and Wrubel (1989:54) give clarity to the meaning of 'situation'.

> *Situated freedom recognizes that the person is no longer viewed as freely choosing all actions all the time. People are either radically free or unfree. Radical freedom is the modern view that people can*

> *choose all their meanings [and actions] all the time. But this view ignores that the choice of meanings is predicated on the meanings [and actions] available to the person's own background, culture and language.*

The holistic practitioner is mindful of the person's situated meaning in making decisions. What may seem rationale and most appropriate to the practitioner may not be so for the person due to their social situation. People do not live in a vacuum; they have prejudices and beliefs honed by socialisation and experience, and being members of cultural and social communities. Within these communities, people have networks of relationships and roles with other people most notably within their own family. Through dialogue the holistic practitioner comes to appreciate the person's situated meaning that can be accepted or confronted as appropriate.

WORKING WITH RELATIONSHIP

Working with is developing a negotiated on-going relationship with the person towards enabling them to meet their needs on the basis of mutual understanding. It is a stark contrast with a task approach to care where the practitioner views the patient as a series of tasks to be done 'to', 'for' or 'at' the patient on a time schedule (Alfano 1971).

Whilst the holistic practitioner always intends to work with the person they are always mindful of the person's situation (as noted above). Hence care is negotiated as a *lived dialogue* based on mutual understanding appropriate to the person's capacity to respond with the person. Kramer (1990: 247) notes –

> *The holistic view holds the individual ultimately responsible for health, and individuals are deemed both capable and responsible for choosing experiences that will enhance health. In the holistic view, the health care provider is not is a detached power position in relation to the patient. Rather both are active and committed participants in enhancing growth towards health... whereby health is viewed as active, changing and creative – i.e. continually changing in novel ways.*

Through dialogue, the practitioner does not impose a dominant view but respects the person's autonomy.[5] Dialogue opens a space to explore possibility where participants gain insight and co-create with the practitioner the best decisions and actions to take, often transcending previous horizons for both participants.

In some situations the person's autonomy to negotiate their own care is compromised requiring the practitioner to make judgement as to the person's best interests. The empathic challenge – 'would the person at a later time ratify the judgement as being in their best interests?' (Benjamin and Curtis 1986).

'TUNING IN' OR WAVELENGTH THEORY

In working with the person, the holistic practitioner *tunes* into the person, literally to get on their wavelength of 'who is this person?' Only when the practitioner is in tune with the person can they appreciate the meanings the person gives to their situation and to negotiate with the person (as able) to meet the person's needs. However, *tuning in* is only the beginning. The practitioner must then *flow with* the person's wavelength as it unfolds (Figure 1.3A). Newman (1994, 1999) describes this as synchronicity; a rhythm of relating in a paradigm of wholeness. Movement along the wavelength can be viewed as a dance, each step a caring movement sometimes led by the practitioner and sometimes by the person as appropriate (Johns 2001).

When people experience crisis in their lives due to illness their wave patterns are likely to become chaotic, fluctuating moment by moment in response to what is unfolding. It can feel like surfing the waves!

From a functional perspective, it is easier to make the person fit-in into the practitioner's wavelength, demanding conformity and compliance to the regime (Figure 1.3B). Indeed this is the 'normal' unreflective stance where the person as a patient is expected to behave with risk of being labelled difficult if non-compliant. Thus the practitioner fails to see the person and cannot be available to the person.

(a)

Synchronicity with the person's wave length

Person's wavelength

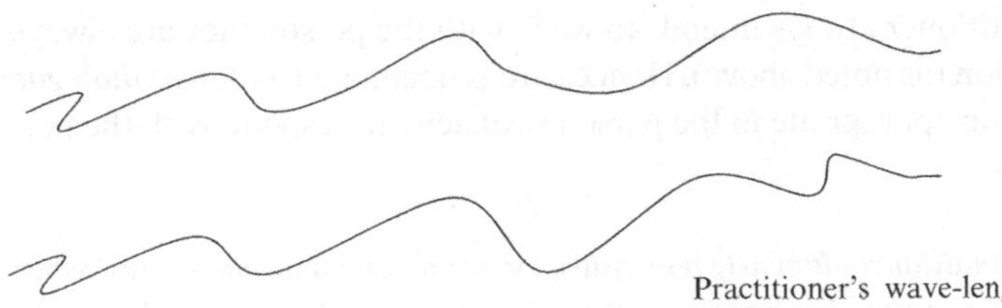

Practitioner's wave-length

FIGURE 1.3A Synchronicity with the person's wave length

(b)

Non-synchronicity with patient's wavelength

Patient's wave-length

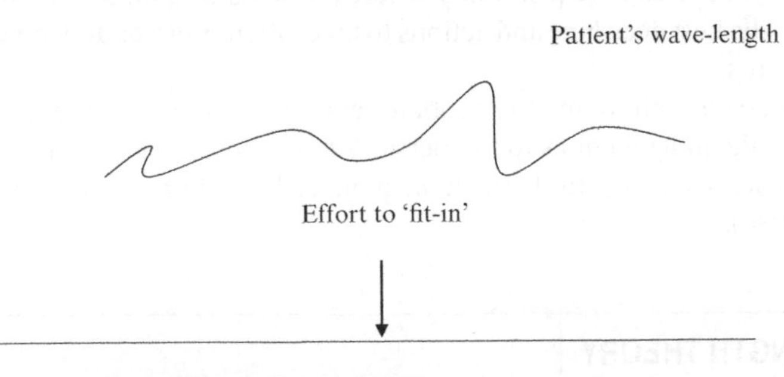

practitioner's wave-length

FIGURE 1.3B Non-synchronicity with patient's wavelength

BEING FULLY PRESENT

The practitioner can easily bring self fully present to the moment by using the breath to clear away distraction and 'bring the mind home'. In the poem 'Naomi' I am mindful of being 'fully present' to her.

Naomi[6]
Pausing at her door
Using my breath to bring myself fully present.
91 years old, never had a thing wrong until this.
This small lady looks up at me
wearing delicate red lipstick
Such thin legs
The football stomach looks incongruous
The ascites being drained.
Had her lungs done a while ago
Ovarian cancer.
I sit
I am in no hurry
And now she can see my face more clearly
rather than my belly.
I hold her hand
Blackwolf and Gina Jones words come to mind
Touch is the harmonic healing the grieving spirit craves
A gentle touch on the back, the shoulder, the head, the hand
Tells the receiver more than what can be expressed.
I have often dwelt upon these words with intent
to communicate she is not alone,
to help her find ease amongst the chaos.
She tries to be rationale
'I've had a good life, the last 20 without my husband surrounded by a good family'.
She tries the brave face
but underneath her suffering ripples.
A nurse pops in to check her drainage tap.
No sense that she might disturb the flow.
Tasks to be done!
Naomi declines the offered therapy.
She has found a comfortable position
as if that position is precarious.
She squeezes my hand and thanks me for my attention.
You never know what to expect when you move into a patient's room.
Simply to be present in the moment,
open to the possibility, in no rush to move on.

PROFESSIONAL INVOLVEMENT (BALANCING CONCERN AND POISE)

As noted within the Being Available Template, concern is a feeling that the person matters to the practitioner. The person will easily discern the extent the practitioner is concerned simply through their manner and sense of presence. Without concern, there can be no genuine relationship. Benner and Wrubel (1989:86–7) note –

Concern is a way of being involved in one's world. Concern describes a phenomenological relationship wherein the world is apprehended directly in terms of its meaning for the self and the things that matter to us.

However, the practitioner is not a robot who can turn 'concern' on when considered necessary as if a tool to be applied. Rather concern is an ontological way of being in the world. Concern may not be easy given the practitioner's socialisation as reflected in Roger's comment (Chapter 8) –

The Burford cues open the tap on feelings that prior to working at Burford had not been an issue simply because I had kept an emotional distance from patients. This was no longer the case. Now 'who I am as a person' was primary in the care I gave.

Roger's comment reflects he had been socialised to be detached necessary to maintain a 'professional distance' from patients. As Menzies-Lyth (1988) notes –

The core of the anxiety situation for the nurse lies in her relationship with the patient. The closer and more concentrated this relationship, the more the nurse is likely to experience this anxiety. A necessary psychological task for the entrant into any profession that works with people is the development of adequate professional detachment.

Professional detachment inevitably results in not seeing persons as suffering human beings but rather as objects of care to do things to, reinforced by a task approach to care designed to reduce the patient into parts. Hence the nurse is protected from the fall-out of suffering. Of course nurses do feel the patient's suffering and suffer more because it has not been acknowledged as nursing work (James 1989). Experiencing anxiety the practitioner looks away.

Be inspired by the words of Blackwolf and Gina Jones (1996:183–4) –

Uncomfortable with the griever's uncertainty about life, deep sadness, encounter with death and changed self, we turn away when we are needed most. Look at times when, perhaps you have turned away. What were you avoiding? Most likely it was your own uncertainty, your own sadness, your own changes, your own mortality. In order to be comfortable with the uncomfortable, you need to confront your life issues. Take this time to look at your life. How do you view death? How do you view life? Take the time to answer these two questions. They are the most important questions you will ever have to face... your physical presence reassures the griever that life is still a familiar scene. The griever needs your presence more than words. Your presence gives a sense of order in the world that has been turned upside down. Your presence offers peace and comfort. Your presence connects the griever to the world. Connection is needed more than ever.

Blackwolf uses words such as 'presence' and 'connection', words that imply *professional involvement*. Professional detachment is incompatible with holistic practice. To be professionally involved practitioners need to develop poise (as noted in the being available template) to enable them to manage their anxiety aroused by such involvement – the ability to know and manage self within relationship. This ability can be effectively developed within the therapeutic team through the challenge and support of guided reflection.[7]

Practitioners (not being robots) have concerns of their own to deal with if they are to be fully available to the person. Hence a key element to being a holistic practitioner is to be aware of one's own concerns, how these may interfere with concern for the person and working towards shifting any interfering concerns towards positive concern. One concern is concern itself. It sets up expectations that the practitioner will be concerned and with it the vulnerability that entails. Hence concern is balanced with poise – the ability to know and manage one's feelings so they do not interfere with being available to the person.

Holism is enabling the practitioner to be authentic, freedom from needing to conform to some stereotype of the 'ideal' nurse whereby they hide behind a veil of detachment viewing the patient as an object to do things to. Jourard (1971) considered that putting on a nurse's uniform is putting on a stereotype to hide behind.

Yet freedom has a price. It requires engagement with the person and the risk of over-involvement when practitioners lack the ability to manage themselves. They can get drawn into the web of the person's suffering, taking on board their suffering as their own. Practitioners' feelings become entangled making it difficult to stand back and see the situation for what it is. As Benner and Wrubel (1989:375–6) point out –

> *It is an art to know what one can offer in a situation without becoming over-extended or assuming more responsibility for the situation than necessary.*

The difficulty nurses have with feelings reflects the lack of personal development within nurse training and work environments that do not encourage emotional work. It is as if nurses are expected to avoid engaging with emotional work.

Taylor (1992:1042) noted the way nurses had been dispossessed of –

> *Their essential humanness as human beings and as people by emphasizing their professional roles and responsibilities.*

Taylor draws attention to the fact that nurses are human too and, as such, are vulnerable to the same issues that face their patients and families. The lack of recognition of humaneness in nursing thought a focus on roles and responsibilities has led practitioners to strive to be something they were clearly struggling to cope with. Taylor noted that practitioners didn't recognise or understand their own ordinariness as human beings. Consequently, they became alienated from themselves in their efforts to cope with and live with the contradictions in their lives. Jourard (1971) notes that such 'striving' damages 'the self' and reinforces the need to cope in a downward spiral of self-destruction towards burnout (see Chapter 2).

LIFTING ENERGY

Concern is a lifting energy that radiates from holistic practitioners that literally lifts other people into a greater sense of well-being. It makes people feel good and eases suffering. As Rael (1993:88–9) writes –

What is interesting about this lifting energy is that when it happens to us, it also happens to other people who are also being lifted to the next level [and] when we began to lift ourselves from where were before to a higher place, something dramatic happens in our lives.

Lifting energy is infectious and radiates through people. Readers will know from their own experience how some people lift you whilst others drain your energy. The last thing a suffering person needs is being cared for someone who drains their energy, for example a practitioner who treats you in an unconcerned way as if you were some object. You know you enjoy working with some colleagues rather than others, especially those colleagues who act as if they are not concerned about people. It is as if they are toxic and contaminate the collective caring environment.

Lifting energy is available to everyone by holding lifting intent and bringing self fully present to the moment using the breath. It is a vital aspect of being a holistic practitioner.

ENABLING GROWTH

Enabling the growth of the other is the essence of caring. Mayeroff (1971: 1) opens the text of 'On caring' – 'To care for another person, in the most significant sense, is to help him grow and actualize himself'.

The holistic practitioner is mindful of enabling the person to grow through the health-illness experience to expand their horizons of health and find a healthier pattern of living. Growth is to fulfil one's human potential whatever that might mean for the person (Maslow 1968). Every moment is the opportunity to grow for both the person *and for self*. Growth is not a one-way street!

Newman (1994) illuminates how suffering creates the opportunity to stand back and take stock of self, especially if suffering is life threatening. Forced out of their complacency, the person may question the very essence of their existence and the things that are really important. Growth is learning new ways of organising self that is conducive with health. However, growth can be difficult for people who are locked into ways of living that are not easily shifted for whatever reason.

JOURNEYING WITH THE PERSON

Holistic practice is journeying with the person extending over time no matter how long or short that journey is, perhaps just a day or two or perhaps extending over weeks. It informs the person that they are not alone, that a practitioner is always available for whatever reason.

The sense of journeying and dwelling with the person is metaphorically captured through the poem 'The Heron and the tree'.

The heron and the tree[8]

Each day we dwell beneath the small tree
That stands outside your window
To witness the change of colour
From green to yellows and reds
And then brown to mark the leaf's descent into the earth.
Each day fewer leaves
Were attached to the tree's life
Reflecting Autumn's time for death
Within the cycle of life.

In the shade of the tree sat Heron
As if a guide who waited patiently
To guide your journey
From this dimension of life to the next.

I know Heron brought you comfort
Even a sense of stillness
In those poignant moments
When fear gripped the raw edge of emotion.

Some days Heron would catch a leaf
Or two as it fell from the tired tree
Damp with rain the leaf held fast
As if reluctant to let go.

The leaves are a symbol of life
Each day a few less leaves
Until the last time I sat with you
Just one or two clung tenaciously to life.

Reluctant to let go
As if each falling leaf was a countdown
To that inevitable moment
When you breath would cease.

Yet you did let go
In peace
Surrounded by your family
to melt into the divine light.

The poem reflects holistic practice as a form of aesthetic expression (Wainwright 2000) more than technical expression. Put another way, holistic practice is grounded in the human-human encounter of being with others rather than doing to others. This enhances its professional identity and status. After all do practitioners really want to be technicians or do they want to truly care?

I have endeavoured to unwrap the essential nature of holistic practice as stated in the Burford hospital vision. Through reflection on experience towards realising holism as a lived reality, practitioners come to explore and find meaning in these words and expertise in living them (see Chapter 6).

THE INTERNAL ENVIRONMENT OF PRACTICE

The internal environment of practice is concerned with the pattern of relationships between all staff. To support holistic practice it is essential to create the *'Therapeutic team'* whereby practitioners are mutually available to each other in ways that mirror practitioners being available to persons. It requires establishing and sustaining collaborative and dialogical ways of working together based on shared purpose, respect and collective responsibility. This has particular significance with respect to primary nursing as the system for organising the delivery of practice due to the relative autonomy of primary nurses (see Chapter 5). It also necessitates a collaborative type of leadership and management of the hospital (see Chapter 2) through its organisational systems.

SOCIAL VIABILITY (THE EXTERNAL ENVIRONMENT OF CARE)

Social utility (Johnson 1974) concerns the role of the practice setting in responding to and influencing societal expectations, and wider professional issues such as research and teaching. It challenges practitioners to look beyond the immediate context of the practice setting towards considering its wider social and professional responsibility.

Johnson identified three strands of social utility:

1. Social congruence is based on the extent to which decisions and actions fulfil social expectations
2. Social significance is determined by the extent to which actions based on the model make a difference to patient outcomes
3. Social utility is determined by the extent to which clear directions for practice, education and research is provided.

SOCIAL CONGRUENCE

At Burford I attended monthly meetings of the Friends of the hospital to promote and discuss Burford's role within the Community, listening to the public's views on health care practice and to influence their thoughts about practice at the hospital.

Consider – how does the local community view the most appropriate use of our beds? Should a quota of beds be set aside for respite care? Should terminally ill patients take priority considering the nearest hospice is 16 miles away?

It was also vital to establish collaborative relationships with the various GP practices that serviced the Burford beds. The GPs were not involved in constructing the vision as being outside the hospital and yet their influence on practice had always been significant. Hence it was important to get them onside with the idea of holistic practice. Pearson had already challenged medical domination of Burford's practice with claiming nursing beds. This was divisive according to the GPs. Hence I realigned the beds as 'patient beds' where admission was negotiated.

Burford hospital exists within a larger Health care Trust with its own expectations on Burford's practice. Hence social congruence always has this political and cultural edge.

SOCIAL SIGNIFICANCE

The proof is in the pudding so to speak. The Burford vision clearly sets out its holistic intention. Implicit within this intent is the perception that holistic practice will make a difference to patient outcomes. The evidence for this lies within practitioner reflexive accounts in recorded guided reflection sessions (Johns 1998). It is also evidenced in the practitioner accounts within this book.

Asserting a holistic vision lifts the significance of nursing and caring into focus. In doing so, it explicitly challenges a health care culture that has not valued nursing or caring. As Watson (1988:33) notes

Caring values of nurses and nursing have been submerged. Nursing and society are therefore, in a critical condition today in sustaining human care ideals and a caring ideology in practice. The

> *human care role is threatened by increased medical technology, bureaucratic-managerial institutional constraints in a nuclear age society. At the same time there has been a proliferation of curing and radical treatments cure techniques often without regard to costs.*

Watson wrote these words 34 years ago. Has anything changed? I sense it is much the same mentality today that dominates health care culture. Hence holistic practice is confrontational and political.

SOCIAL UTILITY

Being an acknowledged Nursing Development Unit, Burford had a responsibility for developing its clinical practice – exemplified by the development of the Burford NDU model and sharing its developments with the wider professional world through its teaching programme, publications and conferences. The very nature of reflective practice turns all practitioners into researchers, inquiring into their own performance and holistic practice. Learning through reflection is reflexive – it develops personal knowing (or personal mastery) that informs future practice in an endless cycle of becoming. Of course, not all practice settings are nursing development units, yet we had no additional resources because of our status. Additional resources were earned through the teaching programme.

NEXT STEP

To reiterate, a vision gives meaning and purpose to practice, challenging the practitioners to collectively work towards realising the vision as a lived reality. However, this requires a strong collective commitment, as practitioners will inevitably stumble across barriers embedded within the organisation and embodied within self. In Chapter 2 I explore systems to facilitate realising holistic practice.

Listen to Blackwolf's drum beat...
Believe in the vision of you
Practice the vision
Become the vision
(Blackwolf and Gina Jones 1996:47)

NOTES

1 'Felt need' is a step within Ottaway's change management strategy [see Chapter 2].

2 This quote is taken from Watson's 1988 book. A revised version was published in 2007.

3 I have made explicit the attribute of clearing the mind from distraction from the previous template.

4 Concern for the person is not compassion. Compassion literally means 'to suffer together'. The holistic practitioner acknowledges the other's suffering yet does not absorb that suffering as their own.see https//:greatergood.berkeley.edu

5 Seedhouse considers that respecting the person's autonomy is the highest ethical principle.Seedhouse D (1988) *Ethics: the heart of healthcare.* Wiley, Chichester.

6 This poem was previously published in Johns C (2022) 'Reflection on not giving a therapy': weaving narrative through prose poetry. In

Becoming a reflective practitioner (sixth edition) (Ed. C Johns) Wiley Blackwell, Oxford.

7 The exemplars of guided reflection in Chapter 6 illustrate this development.

8 This poem was first published in Johns (2006) *Engaging reflection in practice*. Blackwell Publishing, Oxford.

REFERENCES

Alfano G (1971) Healing or caretaking – which will it be? *Nursing Clinics of North America* 6(2); 273–80.

Benjamin M and Curtis J (1986) *Ethics in nursing* (second edition) Oxford University Press, New York.

Benner P and Wrubel J (1989) *The primacy of caring*. Addison-Wesley, Menlo Park.

Blackwolf J and Jones G (1996) *Earth dance drum*. Commune-E-Key, Salt lake City.

Carper B (1978) Fundamental patterns of knowing in nursing. *Advances in Nursing Science* 1(1); 13–23.

Dewey J (1933) *How we think*. J C Heath, Boston.

Hall L (1964) Nursing– what is it? *Canadian Nurse* 60(2): 150–4.

James N (1989) Emotional labour: skill and work in the social regulation of feelings. *Sociological Review* 37(1); 15–42.

Johns C (1998) *Becoming a reflective practitioner through guided reflection*. PhD thesis. The Open University, Milton Keynes.

Johns C (2001) The caring dance. *Complementary Therapies in Nursing and Midwifery* 7(1); 8–12.

Johns C (2004) *Becoming a reflective practitioner* (second edition) Blackwell Publishing, Oxford p48–50.

Johns C (2022) Framing insights. In *Becoming a reflective practitioner* (sixthedition) (Ed. C Johns) Wiley Blackwell, oxford p52–58.

Johnson D (1974) Development of theory: a requisite for nursing as a primary health profession. *Nursing Research* 23(5); 3373–7.

Jourard S (1971) *The transparent self*. Van Nostrand, New York.

Kramer MK (1990) Holistic nursing: implications for knowledge development and utilization. In *The nursing profession: turning points* (Ed. N Chaska) C V Mosby, St Louis.

Maslow A H (1968) Toward a psychology of being. Van Nostrand, New York.

Mayeroff M (1971) *On caring*. Harper Perennial, New York.

McCormack B, McCance T, and Martin S (2021) What is person-centredness? In *Fundamentals of person-centred healthcare practice: a guide for healthcare students* (Eds. B McCormack, T McCance, C Bulley, D Brown, A McMillan, and S Martin) Wiley Blackwell, Oxford.

Menzies-Lyth I (1988) A case study in the functioning of social systems as a defence against anxiety. In *Containing anxiety in institutions: Selected essays*. Free Association Books, London.

Neuman B (1980) The Betty Neuman health care systems model: A total person approach to patient problems. In J P Riehl & C Roy (Ed.), *Conceptual models for nursing practice* (2nd ed., pp. 119–134). Appleton-Century-Crofts, New York.

Newman M (1994) *Health as expanded consciousness*. National league for Nursing, New York.

Newman M (1999) The rhythm of relating in a paradigm of wholeness. *Image: Journal of Nursing Scholarship* 31(3); 227–30.

Pearson A (1983) *The Clinical Nursing Unit*. Heinemann Medical Books, London.

Rael J (1993) *Being and vibration*. Council Oaks Books, Oklahoma.

Seedhouse D (1988) Ethics in healthcare. Wiley, Chichester.

Senge P (1990) *The fifth discipline: the art and practice of the learning organization*. Century Business, London.

Taylor B (1992) From helper to human: a reconceptualisation of the nurse as a person. *Journal of Advanced Nursing* 17; 1042–9.

Wainwright P (2000) Towards an aesthetic of nursing. *Journal of Advanced Nursing* 32(3); 750–5.

Watson J (1988) *Nursing: Human Science and Human care*. a theory of nursing. National League for Nursing, New York.

Watson J (1990) Caring knowledge and informed moral passion. *Advances in Nursing Science* 13(1); 15–24.

Setting Out the Burford NDU Model

CHAPTER 2

Christopher Johns

In Chapter 1 I set out constructing a vision for practice as the foundation for holistic practice. In this chapter I explore the systems and organisational culture of the Burford NDU holistic model designed to enable the vision to become realised within everyday practice. Whilst an individual practitioner can hold holistic intent they will inevitably struggle to succeed alone without the support of like-minded colleagues and an enabling practice environment. Holistic practice requires the whole team.

MODELS OF NURSING

The Burford NDU holistic model was constructed at a time when models of nursing were in vogue. Most models were derived from the USA. They tended to be written in a complex theoretical language that wasn't easy for practitioners to discern their practical value beyond broad ideas such as self-care, adaption etc. As Miller (1985:423) remarked

> *Many nursing theories and models are so abstract and so complex that it is virtually impossible to see their relevance to practice.*

More practical and widely adopted in the UK was the 'Activities of Living' model devised by Roper, Tierney and Logan (1980). Luker (1988) noted that –

> *The advantage of models of nursing based on activities of living is that they are easy to understand and fit in with the personal values systems of many nurses.*

Burford had chosen to utilise this model. Pearson (1983:53) considered that the Roper, Logan and Tierney model –

> *Speaks to nurses in language which is familiar and related to nursing in this country and hence its greatest advantage then is its ability to convey meaning to clinical nurses.*

Luker and Pearson suggest that practitioners, given the opportunity, are likely to choose a model that most fits with the functional way they normally practice. Yet, I discerned no meaningful resonance between the Roper, Tierney and Logan model with the Loeb Centre philosophy that Pearson had imported and imposed on Burford practitioners. Any 'imported' model with its built-in assumptions imposes a reality of nursing on practitioners. Practitioners will tend to

Holistic Practice in Healthcare: The Burford NDU Person-centred Model, Second Edition. Edited by Christopher Johns.

accommodate the model to fit their practice to the model paying lips service to it and continue as they always have done.

As such, it is pertinent to consider whether adopting a model of nursing is merely a conceptually attractive artefact or is it something that can realistically facilitate practitioners to practise more meaningfully in tune with the model's vision?

CHOOSING A MODEL

Take a fresh look and remind yourself of your beliefs about your practice? Are they important to you? Are they truly realised? Models of nursing are explicitly underpinned by a vision and associated assumptions their authors hold concerning the nature of nursing (Meleis 1981). As such, there were only two ways that practitioners can *sensibly* utilise a model as a framework for their practice:

1. By matching their own vision against the model's vision and choosing the model which most resonates.[1]
2. By using their own vision to construct a 'tailor made' model to enable realising their vision as a lived reality such as the Burford NDU model.

Shortly after constructing Burford's vision I brought hospital and community nurses together to reflect on the continued use of the Roper, Tierney and Logan model. The community nurses had not been party to the vision's development yet it was vital to involve them because of their experience in using the model. The community nurses, although managed by me, belonged to a wider professional group of community nurses who were actively trying to develop their unique vision for community nursing across Oxfordshire. I had presented the group with three basic questions:

1. Why do we use the Roper, Tierney and Logan model?
2. What are its relative merits and disadvantages?
3. How does it fit with our newly developed vision for practice?

Prior to this meeting I had undertaken an audit of nursing notes to gain a perspective of how practitioners were recording patient care using the Roper, Tierney and Logan model. The model comprises 12 activities of living. I noted that 'Dying' was never addressed as if dying was excluded as an activity of living. Superficial comments such as 'likes to wear lipstick' characterised 'Expressing sexuality' as if issues around sexuality were taboo or outside the realm of nursing. The eating and drinking box had superficial comments like 'Likes tea in the morning'.

Through reflections of using the model the group concluded:

1. That the model was a reductionist model that split the patient into 12 parts that was the antithesis of holistic or person-centred practice.
2. That the model encouraged practitioners to see the person through the 12 activities of living which narrowed the limit to be creative on seeing the person.
3. That practitioners only filled in boxes that seemed relevant. Whilst this may seem sensible, it created an impression to others that the practitioner had not completed the assessment or did not consider certain activities of living significant.

4. That the notes tended to be superficial and not developed from point of admission and hence had little impact on actual practice.

5. It was difficult to know in which box to record certain information about the patient. This point illustrated how the practitioners tended to fit the patient to the model rather than use the model to see the patient.
   Webb (1986:172) noted –

   Most profound criticisms of nursing models draw attention to problems in using them because they are not spelt out in sufficient detail. Several authors in this book have found difficulty in deciding under which heading to enter a particular piece of information.

6. The paucity of written information reflected how primary nurses were not considering the needs of other nurses attempting to follow care as the primary nurses often had this information in their head. This point also suggested how much of nursing care was based on routine that didn't really require notes. In other words it was a poor method for communicating continuity of patient care.[2]

7. The model did not really encourage any focus on social, spiritual or psychological aspects of the person's experience, reflecting how these aspects of being human had been outside the scope of nursing practice from its functional approach.

8. The model did not focus on what the person's illness meant to that person. In fact, the model was felt to be too 'medically focused'.

9. Assessment was generally viewed as something done on admission rather than the foundation for assessing, planning, and evaluating the patient's care through their stay in hospital and discharge.

10. The model was felt to be insensitive and intrusive – peppering the patient with thoughtless questions prompted by each activity of living. In other words it detracted from seeing the whole person. It did not focus on creating a therapeutic relationship with the patient or family.

11. It was felt to be inconsistent with different practitioners viewing the activities of living differently.

As these points indicate, the group agreed the model was inadequate and certainly did not reflect the hospital's newly constructed holistic vision for practice. Roper, Logan and Tierney could no doubt defend their model against these criticisms as largely stemming from a failure of the practitioners to understand its essential nature. What was shocking to the practitioners at this meeting was their own unreflective utilisation and acceptance of the model. It brought home the need to be more mindful and critical of their practice.

JUMPING THE GUN

In preparation for the review meeting I had 'jumped the gun' by drafting a potential assessment strategy to answer the question – 'What information do I need to nurse this person?' The group agreed to pilot these cues (see Chapter 3). Thus the Burford NDU model took root.

THE FIVE SYSTEMS

Five integrated systems were developed to facilitate the realisation of holistic practice. These systems are set against the background of a dynamic learning culture and holistic leadership (Figure 2.1).

Practice settings will initially be attracted to the Burford NDU model because of its holistic vision and its strategy for tuning practitioners into it to gather information. It is the obvious starting point followed by reviewing existing verbal and written communication patterns for its efficacy to communicate holistic practice, and reviewing whether existing systems for organising the delivery of care is the most effective way to deliver holistic practice. Implementing guided reflection is advocated as the system for developing and sustaining practitioners to become holistic practitioners because it enables practitioners to learn through their everyday experiences and become reflective practitioners alongside a system for living and ensuring the quality of holistic practice. These 5 systems are explored through subsequent Chapters 3–7.

Dynamic learning culture

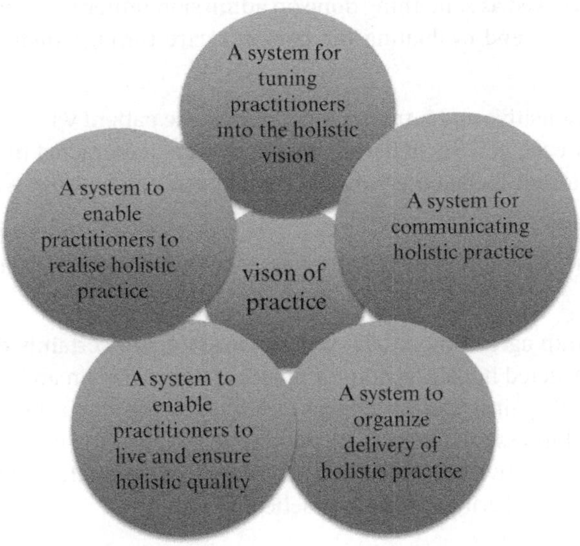

Holistic leadership

FIGURE 2.1 Overview of the five systems and background culture to drive it

A DYNAMIC LEARNING CULTURE

The Burford NDU model is explicitly a dynamic learning culture. By this I mean that its systems are reflexive, always in a dynamic state of becoming, and constantly reflected on through feedback loops for their efficacy to support and enable its vision of holistic practice to be realised and further developed. Holistic practice can never be taken for granted as something known. Every experience becomes an opportunity to learn through dialogue whether as individuals or collectively.

Any practice setting adopting the Burford NDU model will immediately feel a new buzz and energy about the place. The idea of the 'Learning Organization' gives shape to a dynamic learning culture, lifting the idea of learning into practitioners' minds, constantly reminding them that practice and learning is ever static or routine. Everything has meaning and purpose and is in a process of evolution.

Senge (1990:3) defines the Learning Organization as –

> *One where people continually expand their capacities to create the results they truly desire, where new and expansive patterns of thinking are nurtured, where collective aspiration is set free, and where people are continually learning how to learn together.*

Senge identified 5 disciplines that collectively constitute the Learning Organization.

- Vision
- Personal mastery
- Mental models
- Team learning
- Systems thinking

VISION

As I noted in Chapter 1, a valid vision is the foundation of the Burford NDU model. To reiterate, it gives meaning and purpose to everyday practice.

PERSONAL MASTERY

Personal mastery is the ability to be an effective holistic practitioner. It is a continuous process of self-inquiry and self-development through becoming a reflective practitioner. Senge (1990:142) notes –

> *People with a high level of personal mastery live in a continual learning mode, they have a strong sense of purpose, they are deeply inquisitive thus are acutely aware of their ignorance, their incompetence and their growth areas. They are creative and deeply self-confident.*

MENTAL MODELS

Mental models refer to the right attitude to be a holistic practitioner. It is essentially an aspect of personal mastery. Developing mental models towards realising holistic practice will certainly challenge previously held attitudes that are not compatible. This is akin to a seismic paradigm shift from seeing practice that way to seeing it this way.

As Senge (1990:174) notes –

> *New insights fail to get put into practice because they conflict with deeply held internal images of how the world works, images that limit us to familiar ways of thinking and acting.*

TEAM LEARNING

Team learning is a *community of inquiry* whereby practitioners collectively meet to review and develop their practice. It takes personal mastery from an individual issue to a collective issue. Through dialogue[3] practitioners learn to become collaborative, to give and receive valid feedback, take responsibility for both individual and collective practice, deal positively with any conflict and are available to support each other and generally develop the therapeutic team. Learning together practitioners transcend individual horizons of knowing and being.

SYSTEMS THINKING

Systems thinking is the core of the Burford NDU model through its five integrated systems. The idea of *thinking* is to be critically reflective of the adequacy of these systems to support holistic practice. In other words systems must be fit for purpose rather than organisationally convenient. Systems are everybody's business elevating practitioners into an organisational and political responsibility.

HOLISTIC LEADERSHIP

Leadership is the energy and foresight that drives the five systems and the community of learning. Indeed, such is the significance of leadership that I acknowledged it as the sixth discipline of the learning organisation (Johns 2022). What is needed is a leadership congruent with holistic practice – what can be termed 'holistic' leadership.

The contemporary literature on leadership advocates a transformational or servant-leadership style of leadership, both of which are dialectically opposed to the transactional management prevalent in most public service organisations such as health care trusts despite being advocated by the NHS Forward Review[4] at a time of radical change. Nicholson (2009) wrote –

> *Great clinical leadership is fundamental to this. Sustainable health systems are created when clinical leaders are empowered to bring about transformational change supported by managers who back good ideas, remove blockages to progress and provide support.*

Fine words but what is its reality? Nicholson should say 'driven by leaders' simply because managers are focused on tasks, targets and outcomes not processes and relationships. As Wheatley (1999:164) notes –

> *Management is getting work done through others. The important thing was the work; the 'others' were distractions that needed to be managed into conformity and predictability.*

Transformational leadership is concerned with creating and sustaining a dynamic and moral learning organisation to enable people to grow and realise their potential (Bass 1990). Yet, if organisations are primarily concerned with meeting strategic outcomes or targets, or fiscal security, the moral landscape quickly becomes obscured, the human factor lost in the machine (Johns 2016). Servant-leadership (Greenleaf 1977/2002) advocates leaders being 'of service' and creating 'community', ideas essential to holistic leadership and holistic practice.

Holistic leaders:

1. Perceive the whole picture and the shifting patterns within the whole. Hence nothing is viewed in isolation. Everything is connected enabling the leader to perceive issues proactively (rather than reactively).
2. Hold 'positive regard' towards all staff and are 'of service' to enable others to accomplish what needs to be done through genuine collaborative relationships that invests in all staff to enable them to grow and fulfil their potential to ensure that their highest priority needs are being served.
3. Foster 'community' through dismantling hierarchical structures and control, promoting open relationships and responsibility by all practitioners where respective roles are mutually valued, respected and supported within a 'therapeutic team'.
4. Are visionary with foresight anticipating what is required based on a firm poised foot in everyday reality – hence their ability to point the way forward in terms of both vision and systems for realising that vision and the likely pitfalls along the way.
5. Are mindful of their tension between being a holistic leader yet working in a transactional organisation that impose contradictory expectations and the consequential culture shift required to accommodate holistic leadership.
6. Enable others to become servant-leaders.
7. Create and drive the learning organisation through feedback loops to ensure systems are adequate to facilitate holistic practice.
8. Has a high profile presence within the practice area to influence practice through observation, dialogue and participation (I maintained working two days a week in an associate nurse role).[5]

CHANGE MANAGEMENT

A key task of leadership is to engender a culture of inquiry and facilitate the necessary shift of culture to realise holistic practice. Holistic practice is the strange attractor around which systems are created. As Wheatley (1999:132) notes – 'By far the most powerful force of attraction in organizations and in our individual lives is meaning.'

Meaning is created by the holistic vision Letting go of the need to control things creates a culture of creativity and possibility. Table 2.1 sets out the necessary culture shift to realise holistic practice. On a rational level this shift may seem straightforward – 'Yes – we want holistic practice'. However, holistic practice is not a technology that can rationally be put in place. It is a way of being and knowing that has a significant impact on practitioners. Hence the change agent must consider barriers to rationale change if shifting to holistic practice is to be successful. These barriers are embodiment, tradition and authority (Fay 1987). Over time practitioners have embodied 'who they are' as a practitioner, instilled into them from training and through subsequent experience. As such, they are able to go about their practice without much thought, as if the body knows what to do. Tradition sets out 'what we do around here' governed by formal and informal rules and the status quo. Change inevitably 'rocks the boat' causing waves that disturb the normal pattern of practice. Authority reflects normal power patterns within the organisation that, like tradition, will inevitably be challenged with a shift to a holistic culture. Practitioners are expected to act according to their place authority puts them in. The collapse of hierarchical management patterns will inevitably open 'a can of worms' as practitioners squirm to find and learn their new place within the system.

Table 2.1 Cultural shift necessary to accommodate holistic practice

→	
Functional approach with emphasis of doing 'to', 'for', or 'at' the patient.	Holistic approach with its emphasis on *working with* the person in relationship.
A stance of Professional detachment from patients.	A stance of professional involvement with persons.
Reductionist approach that views the patient as a series of problems to fix following the medical model.	Holistic approach that views the person as a 'whole' suffering person needing assistance to meet their health-illness-life needs.
Transactional hospital management driven by top-down approach to control all aspects of practice governed by achieving targets.	Holistic leadership as being *of service* to enable others to take responsibility and succeed with focus on process (where outcomes naturally flow).
Harmonious team.	Therapeutic team (see Chapter 5).
Authoritative patterns of communication (non-reflexive and non-dialogical) and nursing process.	Dialogical communication and reflexive narratives (see Chapter 4).
Practice is learnt through applying theory (e.g. study days).	Practice is learnt through reflection-on-experience (see Chapter 6).
Quality is primarily measured by external agency.	Quality is primarily lived and monitored through internal processes (see Chapters 6 and 7).
Practice is generally 'non-reflective' and 'normal', reactive to any disturbance to its smooth running, and where change is viewed as threatening.	Practice is reflective and proactive whereby all aspects of practice are viewed as problematic as an opportunity for practice development.
Change is overly concerned with maintaining the status quo – hence change is accommodated to fit the existing culture.	Change is acknowledged as chaotic towards enabling the vision of practice to become a lived reality.

Thus to shift culture requires a process of reflection, unlearning and relearning.

The practitioner is primed to identify and challenge these barriers through the MSR (Appendix 2) (see Chapter 6). Perhaps the most difficult aspect of the necessary culture shift is moving from a traditional functional task approach to care in the shadow of the prevailing medical model that reduces people to patients with symptoms to diagnose and treat. The medical model stems from a capitalist conception of health care whereby people are given permission to be ill and not to work in exchange for suspending normal rights to become a patient who is passive and compliant with treatment (Parsons 1951).

With the rise of consumerism and human rights, the medical model has undoubtedly weakened. Doctors have discarded their white coats of patriarchal authority. People now expect to consulted as to decisions about their health and be treated as a human being with empathy, respect and dignity.[6] Indeed, 'the patient's experience' is one marker in the CQC assessment of quality care. Organisations proudly display their 'investor in people' labels.

To drive the culture shift, the leader will need to speak two languages simultaneously: one to promote a culture of holistic practice alongside a language that conforms to wider organisational expectations whilst at the same time undermining this language towards enabling the wider organisation to speak the new language and shift its own expectations.

You might say that's a tough task given the dominating unreflective and anxious nature of the transactional organisation with its hierarchical and bureaucratic structure with its focus on targets rather than the culture of caring practice (Johns 2016). Yet the organisation has an Achilles heel reflected in their vision statements. For example, Royal Devon Healthcare Trust in their 'about us' information they state:

> *We will create a culture which retains, develops, supports and attracts people to work as part of a team to deliver patient centred care.*
>
> *We will embrace new technologies and ways of working to deliver the best possible care and to enable people to stay well. (Royal Devon nhs.uk)*

They subscribe to a 'culture' and 'patient-centred care' and delivering 'the best possible care' and 'enable people' – the language of leadership and holistic practice.

Interestingly they term their human resource director as Chief People officer, suggesting an emphasis on people rather than resources. Their words reflect a shifting organisational culture perhaps fuelled by the expectations of the CQC to become more person-centred towards both patients and staff, squaring the equation that if you want staff to care for patients as people then you must care for staff as people.

The leader knows how to prick the Achilles heel.

However, in my experience, such visions do not profoundly influence practice for reasons the leader/change agent needs to be cognisant. Firstly, they go against the grain of a predominantly task and routine approach to practice. Practitioners do not think in terms of values. Secondly, vision statements are often written in vague rhetoric by someone possibly years ago, pinned on office walls covered by layers of organisational memos or buried away in a policy file. The rhetoric is often grounded in caring clichés such as 'we give individualised care' that is contradicted by even the most casual observation of practice. Hence they are not owned by practitioners and have nothing to do with the reality of everyday practice.

CHANGE STRATEGY

Ottaway's change strategy (1978) 'to implement new norms, new styles and new environment in the work organization' offers an ideal change strategy model to guide change because of its explicit focus on culture shift (and shock). Without this explicit focus on leading change the Burford NDU model is at risk, as with other innovations, of being distorted to fit the existing culture whereby limiting its impact (Latimer 1995).

Ottaway set out the basic characteristics deemed necessary for the effectiveness of this change strategy and addressed in contracting a change relationship (see Table 2.2).

Table 2.2 Ottaway's managing change strategy

Characteristic	Activity
Creating felt need	The leader inquires into current practice, disturbing the taken for granted, challenging practitioner beliefs about the nature of practice, whilst, at the same time, suggesting and influencing the need to construct a new vision of practice grounded in their collective beliefs as the basis for future practice.
Bottom up (as opposed to top-down)	To involve all practitioners in the change process acknowledging that practitioners own their practice and the leadership role is to enable them to realise change based on the new vision of practice. This involvement flattens the hierarchy towards promoting collaborative relationships between all staff (see Table 2.1).
'Tailor made'	Every stage of implementing the Burford model is discussed and agreed with practitioners to 'fit' the Burford environment.
Training as part of the change process	Establishing the system for continuous practitioner development (guided reflection) contracted to enable practitioners to develop the necessary personal mastery to become effective holistic practitioners (see Chapter 6).
Reinforcing new norms/ evaluating process	Feedback mechanisms are established to constantly review and evaluate the impact of implementing the Burford model notably through establishing the *team learning* culture and guided reflection asking: • Do practitioners live the vision effectively? • Are the Burford systems effective in supporting practitioners and ensuring quality of care? • Is leadership fit for purpose? In other words everything is under scrutiny and nothing taken for granted.
Pilot site (testing the water)	Implementing the new culture to other sites in the security that necessary issues have been worked through effectively whilst acknowledging that new sites need to develop effective leadership, to construct their own visions and 'tailor make' the change.

MANAGING RESISTANCE

It is a fact of life that some practitioners may view the idea of constructing a vision a threat, or simply can't be bothered with all that 'nonsense'. Some may even be actively or passively resistant or apathetic, disconnected from caring or so buried deep into a non-reflective but they refuse to be energised.

In leading change, the leader is mindful of the significance of the status quo – that change is not a rationale process but deeply embedded in personal interests. As I discovered at Burford, change had previously been imposed on practitioners through the earlier work of Alan Pearson. In the three years since his departure there had been a 'return to normal' as new norms were not reinforced both from inside and outside the hospital. Old norms and interests had insidiously reasserted themselves. No dynamic learning culture was evident. The GPs had regained their fiefdom from the threat of 'nursing beds'. Hence the idea of new change was perceived as threatening to some staff, notably staff who had worked at Burford for some time and admitted they had only complied with or passively resisted previous change. These practitioners had no real commitment despite agreeing with holistic practice. Indeed they believed their practice was holistic.

The status quo is a social balancing act. Change brings about forces that either promote or resist the envisaged change. The change agent needs to act towards undermining resistant forces and reinforcing positive forces. However, increasing positive forces without addressing resistance tends to increase resistance. Thus change is best done through respectful confrontation in both individual interactions and in community meetings – 'bringing resistance into the open' where it can be seen and responded to whilst acknowledging there is a universal tendency to maintain the status quo by those whose needs are met by it.

Resistance will be reduced when:

- When resisters perceive that respected others support the change.
- That their needs will be better met within a new status quo.
- They feel involved in decision-making, or in other words not as *victims of change*.
- When resisters have the opportunity to experience change with minimal threat.

(Breu and Dracup 1976)

The points reflect the change agent's sensitivity to the impact of change, intent to bring staff alongside the changes with minimal threat through patience and dialogue, and yet maintaining a careful pressure. Indeed, this is a measure of holistic leadership to work with practitioners. The starting point of change is disturbing 'normal practice' to generate felt need to construct the new collective holistic vision and help resistant or apathetic practitioners reconnect to caring. The notion of 'caring' then becomes the resister's Achilles heel' –'if you truly aspire to holistic practice then this needs to change'. The unspoken undertone being 'If you don't aspire to our collective holistic vision – what are you doing here?'

Review meetings were held monthly to reflect on the necessary shift of culture and respond to any emerging difficulties.

BURFORD NDU HOLISTIC MODEL ASSUMPTIONS

Models of nursing have traditionally been underpinned by a set of explicit assumptions. These assumptions are philosophical and theoretical concepts to substantiate the beliefs espoused within the model. They answer the question – 'where do these beliefs and concepts derive from?' As such, they inform and give credibility to the model, notably its integrity and wholeness to adequately guide its vision.

The following assumptions have been revised from the original assumptions (Johns 2004).

Caring in practice is grounded in a valid and holistic vision for practice

1. The core therapeutic of holistic practice is the practitioner being available to the person – a working with relationship to help ease the person's suffering and grow through their health-illness experience to meet and enhance their life needs.
2. Practice is supported by the therapeutic team whereby all staff are available to each other for mutual challenge and support in ways that mirror being available to persons.
3. Practice is a mutual growth process of realisation for both the practitioner and persons.
4. Practice is a dynamic learning organisation driven by a congruent leadership and reflective practices.
5. Practice is a responsive and reflexive form in context with the environment in which it is practiced.
6. Quality is lived as part of everyday practice.
7. Practice at every level is based on dialogue.

Practice is a narrative of practitioners journeying with the person.

NOTES

1 This approach was adopted by practice settings set out in chapters 11–14 and in many other settings.

2 This point is picked up and developed in Chapter 4.

3 See pages 4/1–3 – to explore dialogue as core to the system of communication within the Burford NDU model.

4 https://www.england.nhs.uk/wp-content/uploads/2014/10/5yfv-web.pdf.

5 See Jan Dewing's comments on similar lines in Chapter 10 – Jan replaced me at Burford and continued the work of disseminating the Burford model through Oxford's community hospitals alongside Brendan McCormack.

6 The sense of not being treated as a human being with empathy, respect and dignity are markers of 'holistic practice' – the sense of being reduced to an object is powerfully evidenced in 'People are not numbers to crunch' (Johns C and Rose O 2022).

Johns C and Rose O (2022) 'People are not numbers to crunch': a performance narrative and storyboard. In *Becoming a reflective practitioner* (sixth edition) (Ed. C Johns) Wiley Blackwell, oxford (chapter 12, p.133–142).

Johns C (2014) The importance of empathy: people are not numbers. *British Journal of Cardiac Nursing* 8(10); 466.

REFERENCES

Bass B (1990) From transactional to transformational leadership: learning to share the vision. *Organizational Dynamics [Winter]* 19–31.

Breu C and Dracup K (1976) Implementing nursing research in a critical care setting. *Journal of Nursing Administration* 6(10); 14–17. December.

Fay B (1987) Critical social theory. Polity Press, Cambridge.

Greenleaf R (1977/2002) *Servant-leadership: a journey into the nature of legitimate power and greatness*. Paulist Press, Mahwah, NJ.

Johns C (2004) Becoming a Reflective Practitioner: A Reflective and Holistic Approach to Clinical Nursing, Practice Development and Clinical Supervision (second edition), Wiley Blackwell, Oxford.

Johns C (2016) *Mindful leadership*. Palgrave, London.

Johns C (2022) The learning organization exemplified by the Burford NDU model. In *Becoming a reflective practitioner* (sixth edition) (Ed. C Johns) Wiley Blackwell, Oxford p215–32.

Latimer J (1995) The nursing process re-examined: enrolment and translation. *Journal of Advanced Nursing* 22; 213–20.

Luker K (1988) Do models work? *Nursing Times* 84(5); 27–9.

Meleis A I (1981) *Theoretical nursing: development and progress*. J B Lippincott Company, Philadelphia.

Miller A (1985) The relationship between nursing theory and nursing practice. *Journal of Advanced Nursing* 10(5); 417–24.

Nicholson D (2009) *Implementing the next stage review visions: the quality and productivity challenge*. Memo to all chief executives of NHS healthcare trusts in England [Gateway reference 12396], Department of Health, London.

Ottaway R (1978) A change strategy to implement new norms, new styles and new environment in the work organization. *Personnel Review* 5(1); 13–8.

Pearson A (1983) *The Clinical Nursing Unit*. Heinemann Medical Books, London.

Parsons T (1951) Illness and the role of the physician: a sociological analysis. *American Journal of Orthopsychiatry* 21; 452–60.

Roper N, Logan W W, and Tierney A J (1980) *The elements of nursing*. Churchill Livingstone, Edinburgh.

Senge P (1990) *The fifth discipline: the art and practice of the learning organization*. Century Business, London.

Webb C (1986) Postscript. In *Women's health: using nursing models* (Ed. C Webb) Hodder and Stoughton, Sevenoaks.

Wheatley M (1999) *Leadership and the new science: discovering order in a chaotic world*. Berrett-Koehler, San Francisco.

PART 1

The 5 Systems

System to Tuning Practitioners into the Holistic Vision

CHAPTER 3

Christopher Johns

On meeting a person the holistic practitioner seeks to gather the necessary information to identify the person's needs and to establish a working with relationship (as able) to meet those needs. The focus on gathering information is traditionally termed 'assessment'. However, from a holistic perspective, the idea of 'pattern appreciation' is a more appropriate term as it acknowledges the wholeness of the person (Cowling 2000); that the whole is a pattern reflecting its different parts and movement that the practitioner tunes into and flows with as the person's pattern fluctuates throughout their stay.

The Burford NDU holistic model's approach to pattern appreciation (or assessment) aims to:

- Gather information to appreciate the person's needs (what information do I need to nurse this person?)
- Tune the practitioner into the person from a holistic perspective (to establish the working with relationship)
- Tune into self in context of the person (to be fully present)
- Structure the person's on-going reflexive narrative

Nine reflective cues facilitate these aims:

- Who is this person?
- What meaning does this health/illness experience have for the person?
- How is this person feeling?
- How do I feel about this person?
- How has this event affected their usual life pattern and roles?
- How can I help this person?
- What is important for this person to make their stay in the hospice comfortable?
- What support does this person have in life?
- How does this person view the future for themselves and others?

Holistic Practice in Healthcare: The Burford NDU Person-centred Model, Second Edition. Edited by Christopher Johns.

WHO IS THIS PERSON?

This cue sets the holistic tone and attitude. On meeting a person the holistic practitioner seeks to know the person and connect with the person to establish a working with relationship. It is two people meeting for a specific reason. The holistic practitioner informs the person 'who I am' expressing concern to create a trusting space for the person to reveal their health-illness story as able or with the help of others as appropriate.[1]

Knowing a person is to know them within the context of their wider social and cultural world. The practitioner needs to know the person's social world; their family and friends who are also a focus of care. Knowing the person's cultural world becoming is ever more relevant in a multi-cultural world. Only then can the practitioner can be culturally competent to respect the person's culture. However, this is not enough. The practitioner needs to adopt an attitude of cultural safety, an equitable relationship whereby the practitioner is respectful of the person's identity and being mindful of not imposing their own identity values on the person. It is confronting and overcoming any racial prejudice that interferes with being available to the person.

Appreciating the person's health-illness pattern is developed as a *lived dialogue* Paterson and Zderad 1988:23). Given that persons are essentially self-determining, the idea of a *lived dialogue* is to firstly *listen openly and attentively* to the person's story, and secondly, to dialogue with them in order to understand their experience and the meanings they attribute to that experience as the basis for enabling them [as able] to make best decisions about their health care needs.

WHAT MEANING DOES THIS HEALTH/ILLNESS EXPERIENCE HAVE FOR THE PERSON?

The practitioner seeks to know the person in terms of the reason and meanings the person gives to being here in hospital. The practitioner might say something like 'tell me what has been happening to you?' In listening, the practitioner uses empathy to appreciate what the person might be experiencing. What the person is experiencing is unique for both the person and the practitioner although it is likely the practitioner will have met many people with similar illness. As such, the practitioner suspends imposing any meaning or assumption about what the person is experiencing in order to listen and hear the person's story.

HOW IS THIS PERSON FEELING?

It is likely the person may feel anxious about admission or transfer to the hospital. The practitioner can easily spot anxiety and using cathartic responses such as 'How are you feeling?' or 'I can see you are anxious' or 'This must be tough for you?' – responses intended to enable the person to express any anxiety or fear they may be suffering for whatever reason. As Paterson and Zderad (1976:24) note 'each person comes with feelings aroused by anticipation of the event'.

Simply engaging with the practitioner may itself arouse anxiety. Thus the practitioner's conveying concern and patience will enable the person to relax with their anxiety acknowledged and to some extent relieved. Pursuing information without acknowledging anxiety may heighten anxiety and hinder developing the relationship.

HOW DO I FEEL ABOUT THIS PERSON?

The practitioner may have feelings and emotions about the person, perhaps based on first impressions. Feelings tend to be sub-conscious, yet influencing the practitioner's reaction to the situation. In developing a relationship with the person and their family it is important the practitioner is mindful of their feelings and counters any negative feelings, either those aroused by the person[2] or 'stuff' they are carrying around with them that is likely to blunt their concern for the person and generally interfere with being available to the person, what Corley and Goren (1998) describe as 'the dark side of nursing', a perverse state of affairs that adds rather than alleviates the person's suffering.

Being aware of one's emotions is significant in decision making (Callahan 1988) and emotional issues are most often the trigger for reflection shared in guided reflection (see Chapter 6). Emotional work may not be easy when practitioners have been socialised to maintain personal distance from the patient, not to get involved and such-like. Hence the cue confronts the practitioner with their self. Looking into the mirror so to speak and asking 'Who am I?' This is not necessarily comfortable or easy given that we most likely take ourselves for granted, not particularly mindful of how we present ourselves, oblivious to our attitude, prejudices, and general state of mind.

HOW HAS THIS EVENT AFFECTED THEIR USUAL LIFE PATTERN AND ROLES?

The person's health event may disrupt the person's normal lifestyle. Appreciating the person's lifestyle and expectations enables the person and practitioner to set realistic gaols and how life pattern may be improved whereby the health-illness experience is an opportunity to learn and grow, to shift life pattern to a more healthy wavelength. The very essence of caring is enabling to other to grow (Mayeroff 1971). The practitioner will weigh up aspects of the person's life, yet mindful that the person may not be able to easily shift social norms that determine their lifestyle and relationships. This cue touches on all aspects of the person's life. It may feel very broad for the novice holistic practitioner to grasp in comparison with models of nursing based on activities of living that presents the practitioner with a list as if an aide-memoire. However, it becomes natural to ask 'how has this event affected your normal life?' that will lead into a natural dialogue around aspects such as sleep, eating and drinking, bowel habit, continence, mobility, social activities, and sex. The practitioner listens and picks up the cues to pursue any particular aspect that emerges as significant.

HOW CAN I HELP THIS PERSON?

The practitioner is continuously processing information, identifying need and planning how best to meet this person's needs. Through dialogue, some of the person's needs are already being met. Some needs will be prioritized and others less so until the right moment. Depending on the situation, setting and planning to meet needs is negotiated with the person's active involvement (as able) and with other health care colleagues where necessary. When the person for whatever reason is unable or reluctant to be involved then the practitioner acts considering the person's best interests in collaboration with the person's family and colleagues.

Planning is not set in stone. It will necessarily fluctuate from day to day in response to the unfolding situation and person's wavelength. Assessment, planning, response and evaluation become one fluid moment.

WHAT IS IMPORTANT TO MAKE THE PERSON'S STAY IN HOSPITAL COMFORTABLE?

Coming into hospital disrupts the person's normal life patterns as noted above. The practitioner is concerned to make the person's stay as comfortable as possible notably in considering the environment of care and the particular needs of the person. This is likely to be of significance for persons who suffer chronic illness who have established personal routines for coping and adapting to their lives. Even the most mundane aspects of care cannot be taken for granted as appropriate. Obviously this requires dialogue and often compromise about the extent care can be absolutely personalized.

Issues such as listening to music, not just for enjoyment but appreciating that music can be a therapy to aid healing, reading (do practice settings have books for people to read?), newspapers available or can be ordered and delivered, volunteers who might sit with the person for a chat, and the such-like. There is nothing worse than lying in a hospital bed or alone at home suffering with nothing meaningful to engage the mind and ease suffering.

WHAT SUPPORT DOES THIS PERSON HAVE IN LIFE?

This cue tunes the practitioner into the person's (hopeful) eventual discharge. It draws the person's family into sharper focus. It leads to exploring the adequacy of the person's support and future support needs of both the person and the family. Hence the full range of interventions; giving information, giving advice, confrontation where attitude and behaviour may need shifting, catharsis – enabling the family to express their feelings, catalytic – enabling the family to talk through issues, and support – knowing that the practitioner is on their wavelength available to them.[3]

HOW DOES THIS PERSON VIEW THE FUTURE FOR THEMSELVES AND OTHERS?

This cue prompts the practitioner to view the person's experience along life's continuum; to view it in the context of the person's past experiences and future. The reflective nature of this cue prompts the practitioner to help the person and their family explore the meaning of this hospital experience to imagine the possibilities of the future including death. For example, the practitioner may say quite casually 'how do you see the future?' opening a space for dialogue. In a similar vein the practitioner can ask the family the same question – linked to the previous cue concerning support.

HOPEFULLY THESE NINE CUES MAKE MEANINGFUL SENSE

I have listed the nine cues as a logical and practical way to guide the practitioner to collect holistic information. One cue flows into the next. The cue 'How can I help this person' can be viewed as an underlying cue for the others as each cue provides more information that feeds this action cue. The cue 'How do I feel about this person?' may be challenging. Practitioners may initially shrink away in discomfort unused to looking at themselves or thinking that 'how I feel' is irrelevant. Yet the cue has proved vital for awakening the practitioner's own humanity – that 'who I am' and 'what I feel' is significant in the care I give. I am not a robot (please tick the box when you sign into the computer record)!

The cues are deceptively straightforward and practical. There is no complex language to interpret. They are a heuristic, a means towards an end. They are not boxes to fill in requiring concrete answers. However, I know that when practitioners initially engage with the cues, they are likely to view them as such – a normal response given practitioners' previous experience of using assessment models. With experience and guidance, the practitioner learns to internalise these cues as a natural way of going about their practice. They become second nature and lived moment to moment as a continuous reflective process of paying attention, listening, perception, judgement, action and evaluation. Once internalised, the cues are always 'active', 'lived' through practice as a continuous reflective process of journeying with the person reflected in the person's reflexive narrative (see Chapter 4).

The initial struggle practitioners may have with the cues reflects their thinking and behaviour learn through highly structured approaches to assessment applied in non-critical and non-reflective ways either through previous practice or training. It is as if these assessment strategies have become prisons that limit creativity. Practitioners have been so used to being told what to do they lack confidence to think for themselves and be creative.

In Chapter 4 I explore communication of holistic practice.

NOTES

1 The failure of practitioners to introduce themselves is reflective of a culture that treats persons as objects both patients and practitioners. Without a name 'who are you?' This was very evident in the performance narrative 'People are not numbers to crunch' as referenced in the Preface.

2 There is a considerable literature around the notion of the unpopular patient to support the claim that practitioners may sub-consciously feel negative about patients that influences caring. For example, see Johnson M and Webb C(1995) Rediscovering unpopular patients: the concept of social judgment. *Journal of Advanced Nursing* 21; 466–75.

Kelly M P and May D (1982) Good and bad patients~: a review of the literature and a theoretical critique. *Journal of Advanced Nursing* 7;147–56.

Stockwell F (1972) *The unpopular patient*. RCN, London.

3 These interventions follow John Heron's '*Six-category intervention analysis*' (1975) Human Potential Research Group, University of Surrey, Guildford.

REFERENCES

Callahan S (1988) The role of emotion in decision making. Hastings Center Report 18; 9–14.

Corley M C and Goren S (1998) The dark side of nursing: impact of stigmatizing responses to patient. Scholarly Inquiry for Nursing Practice: An International Journal 12(2); 99–121.

Cowling R (2000) Healing as appreciating wholeness. Advances in Nursing Science 22(3); 16–32.

Mayeroff M (1971) *On caring*. Harper Perennial, New York.

Paterson J G and Zderad L T (1976) *Humanistic nursing*. National league for Nursing, New York.

Paterson J G and Zderad L T (1988) *Humanistic Nursing*. National League of Nursing, New York.

System for Communicating Holistic Practice

CHAPTER 4

Christopher Johns

Communication is the beating heart of holistic practice through *dialogue* with persons and colleagues reflected in written notes to ensure consistent and congruent practice. Communication is *reflexive*, informing practitioners what is currently happening, evaluating what has gone before, and planning to move forward towards meeting the person's needs. To ensure communication is effective practitioners require *communicative competence* from both an oral and written perspective.

DIALOGUE

The key to reflexive communication is dialogue. The word 'dialogue' stems from the Greek dia-logos – 'meaning flowing among and through us, out of which may emerge some new understanding' (Bohm 1996:6).

Dialogue can be with oneself through reflection on a particular experience (for example in writing notes or a reflective journal), with a patient, or with groups of people both informally and formally such as attending a meeting. Isaacs (1993:25) describes dialogue as –

> *a discipline of collective thinking and inquiry, a process for transforming the quality of conversation and, in particular, the thinking that lies beneath it... a movement towards creating a field of genuine meeting and inquiry where people can allow a free flow of meaning and vigorous exploration of the collective background of their thought, their personal pre-dispositions, the nature of their shared attention, and the rigid features of their individual and collective assumptions. As people learn to perceive, inquire into, and allow transformation of the nature and shape of these fields, and the patterns of individual thinking and acting that inform them, they may discover entirely new levels of insight and forge substantive and, at times, dramatic changes in behaviour. As this happens, whole new possibilities for coordinated action develop.*

Isaacs suggests that dialogue is collective inquiry leading to consensus and potential transformation in ways of thinking and responding. In other words communication through dialogue is a constant learning process, the driving factor within the dynamic learning culture.

Holistic Practice in Healthcare: The Burford NDU Person-centred Model, Second Edition. Edited by Christopher Johns.

SIX RULES OF DIALOGUE

Bohm (1996) discerned six rules of dialogue:

1. Commitment to work with others towards consensus for a better world
2. Awareness and suspension of one's own assumptions and prejudices
3. Proprioception of thinking
4. Openness to possibility and free from attachment to ideas
5. Listening with engagement and respect
6. Mutual appreciation of dialogue

Dialogue is always moving towards consensus to realise the collective vision of holistic practice as a lived reality. The emphasis on *moving towards* acknowledges a letting go of attachment to old ideas. Dialogue is listening. I mean listening when practitioners give their full attention to what is being said free from distraction and expectation. Not easy in busy environments when the mind is bombarded by stimuli.

The assessment cue – 'Who is this person' challenges the practitioner to listen to the person's story as the basis for care putting aside their own preconceptions. Do we listen to what we want to hear, or distorting what we hear in order to fit into our own scheme, to confirm our own assumptions? To really listen practitioners must not only know and suspend their assumptions and opinions, but also be aware of the thinking that gave rise to these assumptions in the first place. Where do they arise from, how tenacious do we cling to them? Why do we cling to them? This requires a proprioception of thinking, an awareness of where the mind in the moment. Within the dialogical process there is a shift from problem solving towards acknowledging and resolving paradox that requires thinking about the way people think about things. If practitioners use the same thinking that caused the problem to try and solve the problem they would probably fail. Hence practitioners need to change the way they think in order to view problems differently. Only then can they transform their perspectives to see things differently. Finally it requires that those involved in dialogue have a mutual appreciation of dialogue to ensure it takes place, especially in situations of strong feelings and conflict.

CULTURE SHIFT

However, dialogue is not a natural form of communication. As Isaacs further notes (1993:24) –

> *Most forms of organizational conversation, particularly around tough, complex, or challenging issues lapse into debate (the root of which means 'to beat down'). In debate one side wins and another loses; both parties maintain their certainties, and both suppress deeper inquiry. Debate reflects patterns of power relationships and rivalry, were people jostle for control typified by people lining up to get their point across and win the argument. Very little genuine listening takes place. People partially listen to what they want to hear, seeking feedback to reinforce their position rather than be open to new possibility through dialogue.*

Isaacs suggests that communicating through dialogue is a culture shift from existing patterns of communication. As such, it will probably be a significant challenge for most practices aspiring to holistic practice through implementing the Buford NDU model. When you next attend a meeting, or talk with a colleague, patient or relative, first listen and reflect on the pattern of communication. What do you discern about the nature of this talk considering Isaac's words?

DEVELOPING COMMUNICATIVE COMPETENCE

Dialogue is the core of communicative competence that can only really be learnt through practice and reflection. It is always contextual, depending on the particular situation. It is not something learnt from theory. Learning to dialogue needs intent and perseverance to establish the necessary culture shift and develop dialogical skill.

To give an idea of how group dialogue within a meeting might be developed:

1. Appoint a rule keeper who sets out the basic dialogue rules
2. Each person wishing to speak raises their hand for rule keeper to decide (so not everyone is trying to speak at one).
3. Each speaker picks ups the topic of dialogue from the last person (enabling listening and continuity rather than divergence).
4. Periodically stop and reflect how dialogue is progressing noting any difficulties (keeping on the right track, who is doing all the talking and enabling others to dialogue).
5. At the end of the meeting posing whether consensus been achieved (summarising outcomes).
6. Round robin assessing efficacy of dialogue (what have we learnt about dialogue).
7. Subsequent meetings rotate the rule keeper (dialogue is everybody's responsibility).

CONSTRUCTING VOICE

To dialogue effectively requires the practitioner to develop their constructed voice – a voice that is passionate, informed and assertive. The work of Belenkey et al. (1986) offers a typology of voices towards constructing voice through a number of stages that practitioners can identify with as representing their position and pointing the way forwards.

The five stages are:

- Silence
- Received voice
- Subjective voice
- Procedural voice: the separate and connected voices
- Constructed voice

The silent practitioner has no voice at all. Many practitioners may identify with this 'voice', unable to speak out when necessary to do so, and hence unable to have a say in 'what goes on' or promote holistic practice. It is an impoverished and oppressed voice.

The practitioner with the received voice speaks through the words of others. They have no voice or even thoughts of their own. Again it is an impoverished and oppressed voice.

The practitioner's subjective voice rings with opinions about practice, suggesting underlying beliefs about practice. However these opinions are most often without substance. I have noticed when guiding others through guided reflection that this is the voice that must first be cultivated.

The subjective voice develops into the procedural voice. It has two elements; the separate and connected voices. The separate voice is a voice able to be critical of ideas and theory and how this applies to their practice. The connected voice is empathetic, able to tune into and connect to the experiences of others. Again, based on my experience in enabling practitioners to develop this voice, they are guided to connect with relevant theory and assimilate into practice in relation to the experiences they are reflecting on working with patients. In this way, they develop both the separate and connected voices and synthesise these voices towards developing their constructed voice.

ASSERTIVENESS

However, having a constructed voice does not mean that it is heard or listened to. Belenkey et al (1986:184) with a salutary voice note –

> *Even among women who feel they have found their voice, problems with voice abound. Some women told us, in anger and frustration, how frequently they felt unheard and unheeded. In our society, which values the word of male authority, constructionist women are no more immune to the feeling of being silenced than any other group of women.*

I have experienced practitioner's this anger and frustration so often in guided reflection. Male authority or authority in general is traditional in health care organisations where even women speak like men to impose control over the organisation and manage their anxiety that things run smoothly.[1]

Hence practitioners need to develop an assertive voice – to speak with an informed, empathetic, passionate *and assertive* voice. This involves understanding and chipping away at the barriers that have stifled asserting their voice.

To guide practitioners to develop their assertive voice within the context of the particular situation I developed the assertiveness action ladder [Box 4.1]. Each step of the ladder is a challenge to overcome. Step 6 is like taking a deep breath and plunging in yet suitably prepared through the preceding steps. Yet having plunged in steps 8–10 help the practitioner navigate the interaction. Stage 8 refers to 'staying in adult mode' taken from 'Transactional Analysis theory'. Within transactional organisations those up the hierarchy often speak to those below them when anxious (or confronted by an assertive person) as a critical parent that often reduces the other into either a child or less usually into a competitive parent. The first leads to successful although unsatisfactory communication whilst the other leads to conflict. The key is to be mindful of one's feelings to stay in adult mode with the intention of keeping the other also in adult mode when the situation can be most effectively resolves. To do this it is helpful to have the mindset 'I am as powerful as them' and exposing their own contradictions. Of course, this may prove difficult with the urge to retreat knowing that the situation cannot reach consensus. The others simply don't listen and try to put the practitioner back into place. Step 10 is the 'get-out clause' – that it is OK to yield without the practitioner feeling they have failed without losing face, having made their point. Yet the interaction will leave its mark even though that may not be obvious.

BOX 4.1 THE ASSERTIVENESS ACTION LADDER (JOHNS 2022:46)

10	Treading the fine line between pushing and yielding	'Ok – I know how far to push this without becoming marginalized. Yielding is not a weakness.'
9	Playing the power game	'I am as powerful as them – remind them of their rhetoric to be "person-centred".'
8	Staying in adult mode	'Be mindful and don't let them reduce you into child mode.'
7	Being communicatively skilful	'Yes – I know the most effective responses to use (Heron).'
6	'Just do It'	'Yes – stop prevaricating- just do it!'
5	Creating the optimum conditions to assert self	'Yes – I know the most appropriate and beneficial environment to assert my point of view.'
4	Making a good argument	'Yes – I am suitably informed to make my case.'
3	Authority to assert self	'Yes – I must assert myself to preserve my integrity.'
2	Ethically right to assert self	'Yes – it is necessary and right to assert'
1	Feeling the need to assert self	'I feel frustrated – I must act!'

SIX-CATEGORY INTERVENTION ANALYSIS (HERON 1975)

In step 7 of the assertiveness action ladder I note – 'being communicatively competence' with reference to Heron. Specific communicative techniques such as 'Six Category Intervention Analysis' enable the practitioner to develop communicative competence to structure dialogue. Heron proposes six basic therapeutic interventions that can be either authoritative or facilitative.

Authoritative interventions are:

- *Giving information* – enabling the other to make a rational decision based on information
- *Giving advice* – helping the other see other, better ways of seeing and doing things
- *Confrontation* – challenging the other's restrictive attitudes, beliefs or behaviour

Facilitative interventions are:

- *Being cathartic* – enabling the other to express a difficult emotion so it can be resolved
- *Being catalytic* – enabling the other to talk through an issue
- *Being supportive* – communicating a sense of 'being there' for the other

Heron categorised these interventions as manipulative or perverse where the practitioner abuses the responses to meet their own agenda. From a perverse perspective, confrontation might be used to challenge someone's behaviour because you take it personally and makes you anxious rather like a critical parent to a naughty child – 'Don't do that'. From a therapeutic perspective, confrontation is always person-centred – 'Do you think that is the best way to act?' – suggesting that the way the person's behaviour is not the most effective yet without explicit judgment enabling the person to reflect on their own behaviour.

In working with others, the holistic practitioner considers the most appropriate interventions to suit the situation, moving easily between each response as appropriate.

For example:

1. When an underlying emotion is sensed – the practitioner may use a cathartic response – 'you seem angry?' The intention is to surface and release the underlying emotion so it can be dealt with. At this level practitioners may fear releasing the emotion because they do not know how to respond to it.
2. Having released the emotion, the practitioner may use a catalytic response to help the person talk through the issue with the intention of helping them find meaning in their feelings, and through talking through it, to understand deeper underlying reasons and assumptions for these feelings. In this way the person is helped to convert the released negative energy into positive energy for taking action, relieving stress and knowing what to do.
3. Confrontation may then be used to challenge, yet always within a supportive framework. Confrontation is a subtle rather than direct intervention – for example – 'Can you see other ways of responding?' implicitly suggesting that the practitioner's response was not effective, yet without direct judgement. Confrontation is easier within a trusting relationship because the person is more open to challenge, because they know the practitioner has their best interest at heart.
4. Information can be given to help the person make decisions or frame situations. I am wary of giving advice because it is taking responsibility for the other person. Much better to say 'What options do you have' rather than 'I would do this'. If the practitioner considers it is appropriate to give advice they might say 'I am going to give you advice' and imagine I have a neon warning sign over my head that says 'Giving advice' – to remind me that this is a power intervention and to remind the supervisee to take it with caution.
5. Underlying all these interventions is giving support – communicating the sense of presence being with the person.

Burnard and Morrison (1991) identified that practitioners were generally not skilled at cathartic, catalytic and confrontational responses, and yet these are the very essence of holistic practice, a finding that perhaps indicates the nurse's traditional authoritative attitude towards patients and lack of focus on psychosocial aspects of practice.

COMMUNICATING AT HANDOVER OF CARE (SHIFT REPORT)

When I arrived at Burford, handover of care from one shift to another formally took place in the office. The practitioner handing over care reported relevant information for the practitioner(s) receiving care to continue the patient's planned care. The nurse handing over care rarely used the patient's notes reflecting the traditional oral culture of handover. Receiving nurses rarely asked questions. Nor did the handing over nurse prompt discussion. The report was factual. Often the receiving practitioners would write memos on scraps of paper, which detracted from any discussion about care.

I discussed my observations with these same colleagues, suggesting we move towards a more reflective format with greater emphasis on dialogue to create opportunity for practitioners to reflect on the way practitioners were thinking, feeling and responding to patients. Most practitioners agreed this would be helpful and in tune with the newly created holistic vision for practice. However, practice did not easily change as practitioners were locked into this socialised format of handover.

As such, I challenged the primary and associate nurses to role-model dialogue by revealing their own thoughts and feelings and reflections on care, raising issues for dialogue. By asking 'what do you think?' 'how do you feel about her?' 'Could we approach this differently?' In this way practitioners became involved, their contributions encouraged. Handover became a community of inquiry creating a greater sense of collegiality between practitioners. In enabling sharing of feelings, negative feelings could be challenged by asking – 'why do you think the patient feels that way?' Or 'why do you think she is angry?' As a result, through voicing and understanding, more positive feelings emerged. This did not mean that information was not given but the emphasis had changed. Notes could be read before or after the handover, which led to a further challenge of their adequacy.

BEDSIDE HANDOVER

Sitting around in 'the office' discussing patient care can be deemed inappropriate from a holistic perspective of involving the person and their family in their care (Ward 1988). If practitioners value involving persons in decision-making and evaluation of their care, then it is incumbent on them to create space where this can happen. What better opportunity than by moving the shift report from the office to the patient's bedside? 'Don't sit down nurse it's time for report'! quote Rowe and Perry (1984).

Do persons want to be involved in their care? For many reasons they may resist (Waterworth and Luker 1990, Ashworth and Longmate 1992, Biley 1992, Trnobanski 1994).[2]

We decided to implement bedside handover. Not without some resistance from practitioners who did not feel comfortable outside the office and its concomitant threat to patient confidentiality by disclosing information in public spaces.

The approach to implementing the bedside handover at Burford hospital was written as a protocol [Box 4.2]. Bedside handover enables practitioners to:

- Greet the patient (and family)
- Invite patients to reflect on their care and care planning
- Enable patients to give their perspective
- Make better sense of information having seen and spoken to the patient beforehand before moving into 'the office'

The protocol emphasises written notes as the primary means for communication care rather than the oral handover. Stage 4 refers to patient confidentiality. The standards group penned a standard of care: 'Patients do not have confidential information disclosed about them accidently' (this standard is shown in the following chapter concerned with a system for living and ensuring quality).

BOX 4.2 BEDSIDE HANDOVER PROTOCOL

Stage	Action
1	The nurse who orientates the person/family to the Unit draws attention to the style of communication practised by practitioners with patients (as stated in the Unit booklet), emphasising the patient's right not to be involved in hand-over and for confidentiality/ consent to participate.
2	Times for handover are noted.
3	Hand-over commences with nurses involved visiting the patient at the bedside. This approach is referred to as 'the walk-round'. The intent is to invite patients/ families to reflect on their care.
4	The patient's right to confidentiality during the walk-round as advised by the UKCC (1987) is respected. As such, nurses act to enable the patient's control over the disclosure of information. The nurse leading the walk-round may sensitively cue the patient to prompt disclosure as appropriate (see standard of care on confidentiality).
5	Following the walk-round, the nurses continue the report in the staff room to fill in gaps of information or understanding.
6	The primary means of communicating care is the patient's notes written as narratives (see standard on ensuring continuity, consistency and congruence of care)
7	Following the report, the nurse continuing care assures herself of patient care by continuing the patient's narrative, updating the narrative as necessary.
8	The patient's notes are clearly marked and stored by the patient's bed within the storage bin.[3]

Stage 8 of the protocol refers to storage of the patient's notes. It was decided to store these with each person because we viewed these as belonging to them. This practice challenged practitioners to become mindful of what they write knowing that it might be read by the person and their family. Hence holistic practice is transparent requiring openness and honesty. Without these attributes it is difficult to say you 'work with' the person.

TEAM MEETINGS AND DE-BRIEFING

Each month, community meetings were scheduled for all staff to attend to dialogue about any issues concerning realising holistic practice. These meetings were a significant aspect of team learning where staff could voice and de-brief concerns. This acknowledged that staff experience situations that can be tough and emotional, generally 'de-fusing toxic stuff' (Johns 2022:230).

PERSON'S NOTES: MOVING TO A REFLEXIVE NARRATIVE

The primary form of communicating practice is the *reflexive narrative*. It commences with 'who is this person?' gathering information pertinent to planning and giving care to meet the person's needs and continues throughout the person's stay in hospital and eventual discharge.

Writing narrative engages colleagues in (and using Isaacs's words from above) *collective thinking and inquiry*. It is a process of critically looking back and evaluating what has taken place and considering the way forward.

As Paterson and Zderad (1988:7) note that –

The process of how to describe nursing events entails deliberate, responsible, conscious, aware, non-judgmental existence of the nurse in the situation followed by authentic reflection and description.

Reflexive narrative is a meaningful and practical way that builds on nursing's traditional oral mode of thinking, feeling and communicating about practice (Street 1991). It makes sense because it *tells the story* of journeying with the person towards meeting the person's needs.

Writing narrative is carefully constructed.[4] As such it is most effective when recording information is:

- Concise, or to the point, without waffle.
- Clear without ambiguity so its messages can easily be understood
- Complete without missing information
- Cohesive so all aspects make sense as a whole
- Context of holistic practice as a background

THE NURSING PROCESS RE-EXAMINED: AN HISTORICAL NOTE

Implementing narrative is a shift from previous ways of communicating. Burford practitioners had used the nursing process. On review of its use, practitioners considered the nursing process an inadequate method of planning and communicating patient care. The review concluded that it was illogical to continue to use this format as it was meaningless and time consuming, wasting precious time in busy days. It is logical that all tools used by practitioners should be designed to do the job most effectively. Consider – does a skilled carpenter choose a blunt spoon to chisel wood?

The nursing process had been imposed on practitioners as a rational way to go about assessing, planning, giving and evaluating individualised care. In theory, a practitioner should be able to pick up a care plan and continue the patient's care as a seamless activity, altering it as necessary to reflect the shifting pattern of the patient's care. Yet the rigidity of the care plan makes this difficult to do especially for non-physical aspects of care that do not lend themselves easily to goal setting and evaluation because of their indeterministic human nature. Attempts to do this led to stereotypical responses such as 'reassure' or 'give her time to talk'. Planning physical care is easier because its more concrete nature is amenable to goal setting.

The nursing process later attracted much adverse criticism (Latimer 1990, Howse and Bailey 1992, McElroy et al. 1995, White 1995) confirming our own findings. Although the nursing process was intended to promote individualised care (de la Cuesta 1983), ironically the opposite happened when accommodated into the prevailing UK nursing culture characterised by allegiance to the reductionist medical model that resulted in a minimal or lip-service response to the ideology of individualised care (Latimer 1990). It is easy to see why, because splitting up the patient into problems mirrored the medical model. The nurse could now 'diagnose problems'. Despite its intent to individualise care, it actually encouraged the practitioner to reduce the patient into a neat set of 'problems' that needed fixing.

A VIEW FROM OUTSIDE BURFORD

I gleaned a view of written notes from outside Burford by undertaking a study of the impact of introducing primary nursing in another community hospital (Johns 1989). One practitioner commented 'much of it is just nursing, you don't need to write that down'. This comment reflected the pattern recognition and common sense knowing this practitioner and her colleagues possessed and their struggle to write down what was so patently obvious to them. Another practitioner commented 'patients we know well don't need care planning'.

I asked one primary nurse on her return from holiday if she had read her patient's notes. She responded 'I haven't had time because it's so busy'. Intuitively she had picked up what was necessary through the verbal handover. Auditing the notes bore out these comments. The notes were virtually meaningless and served no practical purpose and had virtually no reference to non-physical aspects of care. However, I sensed that these nurses' intuitive knowing of what to do was not based on appreciating the patient's life pattern but from knowing the patient in terms of their own perspectives. In other words patients did not need care planning because all patients are alike with similar physical needs.

Yet these nurses still felt compelled to write in the notes even though they felt it was meaningless and a waste of time, motivated by an internal censor that if nothing is written then care has not been carried out. The fear is compounded when audit systems are constructed around reviewing patient notes.

ENOUGH IS ENOUGH

Following the review, Burford practitioners agreed the nursing process had serious limitations in being 'fit for purpose'. Audit of the notes revealed the paucity and irrelevance of information recorded. No wonder they felt awkward. But it did illustrate how practitioners become victims of imposed systems – yet surely as professionals they should use their own tools? As Batehup and Evans (1992) exclaimed 'why do we keep this sacred cow?' Why indeed. Things had to change. It was clear that practitioners did not think like the nursing process. In fact it constrained thinking. Most practitioners know this, yet have been unable to move beyond this deeply embedded worldview because the nursing process has come to dominate the way practitioners are forced to conceptualise their practice. Even when practitioners do acknowledge the absurdity of the nursing process they seem powerless to move to more meaningful and practical ways of planning and communicating care reminding me yet again of the passivity and powerlessness of nursing generally.

So I posed to Burford practitioners – what alternative ways are there given our holistic approach eschews any reductionist and deterministic approach to our practice?

The answer was a reflexive narrative and dialogical approach that matched pattern appreciation through the nine reflective cues to gather information (previous chapter).

NURSING DOCUMENTATION

A set of documents was designed [Appendix 1].

- Person narrative – Personal data
- Person narrative – Assessment cues

- Person narrative – Information on admission
- Person narrative – Continuation notes
- Person narrative – Special intervention sheet
- Person narrative – Discharge planning sheet and discharge protocol

These documents are designed to be used flexibly as most meaningful and practical within the on-going narrative.

REGINALD SIMPSON (CALL ME REG)

To give an impression of a reflexive narrative 1 set out my initial narrative working with Reg Simpson [Box 4.3]. I established an initial Special Intervention sheet to give emphasis to his on-going support needs and daughters' anxiety. The list of identified 'problems' can be transferred to a care plan for clarity of communicating information as a check list (see Appendix 2).

Reg was far from satisfied with his first night's sleep so I implemented a sleep visual analogue scale [Sleep VAS][Box 4.4]. Using the Sleep VAS enabled Reg to monitor his satisfaction with sleep. The Sleep VAS was specifically designed for use at Burford as the method to monitor outcome criteria within the sleep standard of care.[5]

BOX 4.3 EXTRACT FROM REG SIMPSON'S REFLEXIVE NARRATIVE

Date	Nursing history	Sig
6/11	Reg was admitted this morning for one week's respite care. He has been attending the day care for the past 4 months (see attached notes). He is 93. He has cancer of the prostate gland with bony spread. He lives alone although his 2 daughters live close by and provide support for him on an on-going basis including ensuring he takes his medication. However, as Reg says 'I'm not managing so well.' He feels very tired and uncoordinated. His pain is well controlled on MST 20mg bd. (see pain chart). He said, 'this morning I got myself in a real mess getting dressed.' He feels he will need more support. His daughters need a break from caring – hence this admission. Reg wears a hearing aid and requires people to speak loudly to hear. He is very philosophical about this admission and indeed about his eventual death. He was tearful when talking about his wife who died 27 years ago. I asked him if he imagined being reunited with her? He laughed and said 'No'. He has no strong faith – 'I think I will simply return to the earth from whence I came.' He still enjoys reading the *Guardian* newspaper, doing crosswords and watching TV. He has been a very keen angler but fears he may lose this – so dependent on help to continue fishing. He enjoys company, chatting – indeed very appreciative of my chat with him, especially talking about philosophical issues. Has worked in a bank all his working life.	cj

(Continued)

BOX 4.3 (CONTINUED)

Date	Nursing history	Sig
	Reg presents with a number of needs (as reflected on his care plan) 1. difficulty with sleep 2. has a catheter which he dislikes but it is working OK. 3. poor appetite – he says he enjoys soups. He says he has lost weight over the past months. However, he takes this in his stride. He enjoyed his soup for lunch and managed some pudding. 4. fatigue, 5. fragile skin – he has a small break on left hand after an accident with his grandson. No other breaks. 6. anxiety about the future support – see SI sheet 7. He is on a wide range of medication for his heart (see list). He also takes an anti-depressant (daughter manages his medication) 8. Symptom management (reliant on daughters for medication). 9. Increasing loss of mobility – he has stopped using his electric scooter at home because he was getting his feet mixed up! He walks with a zimmer frame – in fact walked with one nurse to eat lunch at the communal table. Lacks confidence – physiotherapy referral. 10. He has some lower oedema for which he wears 'tubigrip'. 11. Prone to constipation – monitor with bowel chart	
	Progress/ evaluation record	
7/11	New wound noted on outer side of right leg – he knocked his leg on side of the bed [see SI sheet]. Seen by Maggie (Physiotherapist) – he can walk with one person safely but we do need to encourage his walking but remember he is easily fatigued! He enjoyed a 'jacuzzi bath' this morning. Reg woke as usual at 04.00 this morning and lay restless until breakfast – see SI sheet/ VAS. This afternoon Reg was dozing in his chair as he does at home. He asked me the time. I said 4:00 p.m. He groaned! 'Oh – no, when's dinner time?' He is clearly bored. He structures his day through meal events (even though his appetite is poor). I asked him how the crossword went yesterday – he said "I wasn't in the mood.' I found him the *Telegraph* for today (note – the *Guardian* is ordered for tomorrow). Hazel (care assistant) will help him later with it as he enjoys company. Seen by Dr Webb – he is booked for thyroid function test on Monday. Also a review use of 'sertraline' (antidepressant) – does he need this? Perhaps Reg can go to Day care tomorrow to engage him? [although not his regular day care day].	

BOX 4.4 **MONITORING REG SIMPSON'S SLEEP PATTERN USING SLEEP VISUAL ANALOGUE SCALE [SVAS]**

Sleep VAS	Name	Date
	Reg Simpson	6/11

Complete satisfaction with sleep — No satisfaction with sleep

*<-->

Mark perception on scale

Note factor that influence the mark?

NB: pain, position, hunger, drink, temperature of room, noise, bed, bedclothes, anxiety, emotion, usual sleep pattern, sleeping tablets, full bladder, other?

Reg says he slept worse than he has been doing at home despite maintaining his normal sleep pattern. He felt being in the hospital was OK although it was strange being in another bed – not so comfortable as his bed at home. Comforted by nurse spending time with him in the 'early hours'. No pain

Action – increase night sedation?

Sleep VAS	Name	Date
	Reg Simpson	7/11/

Complete satisfaction with sleep — No satisfaction with sleep

*<-->

Mark perception on scale

Note factor that influence the mark?

NB: pain, position, hunger, drink, temperature of room, noise, bed, bedclothes, anxiety, emotion, usual sleep pattern, sleeping tablets, full bladder, other?

Sedation not increased. Yet Reg seemed more dissatisfied with his sleep than last night. I sat with him and talked about his wife and the prospect of not being able to cope at home anymore. He had half a cup of tea and seemed more settled afterwards.

Sleep VAS	Name	Date
	Reg Simpson	8/11/

Complete satisfaction with sleep — No satisfaction with sleep

*<-->

Mark perception on scale

Note factor that influence the mark?

NB: pain, position, hunger, drink, temperature of room, noise, bed, bedclothes, anxiety, emotion, usual sleep pattern, sleeping tablets, full bladder, other?

Reg more satisfied with his sleep although awake again – he said he enjoyed day care – took his mind off things. I gave him a hand massage and some lavender and he managed to doze for another hour.

SELF-ASSESSMENT

The Burford assessment strategy is easily adaptable for self-assessment to gain information from the family prior to the point of admission for respite care. This is particularly useful if the person being admitted is a poor historian and recognising that it may not be easy for the family to hand over care to another. Dawson (1987) noted that spouses in particular, equated caring duty as a marital responsibility, leading to a strong sense of guilt when the spouse sought respite care. Does this tell the world that the spouse can no longer manage and hence has failed to care? The family may feel anxious that hospital practitioners cannot know the person well enough or feel they have lost control of the caring role. Will the practitioners mess up normal patterns of care creating potential problems after discharge?

Appreciating this scenario of self-assessment enables the family/carer to:

- Set out in detail the person's normal lifestyle pattern
- Feel in control and involved in the care process
- Feel recognised and valued as the main carer
- Have their own needs recognised as a legitimate aspect of 'whole' care
- Identify need for further support.

The carer's assessment becomes the focus for negotiating care. All the 'little things' (Macleod 1994) that the carer feels are important are identified and acknowledged to minimise the risk of the person's and carer's normal lifestyle pattern being disrupted although, at discharge improvements to life style pattern may well have been indentified. Hopefully, the carer can then enjoy her respite break in a more relaxed frame of mind.

CULTURE SHIFT

In Box 4.5 I summarise and contrast the cultural shift moving from the nursing process to reflexive narrative. This is linked to Table 2.1 that set out the broader necessary culture shift to accommodate holistic practice.

BOX 4.5 CULTURE SHIFT FROM NURSING PROCESS TO REFLECTIVE NARRATIVE

Nursing process	Reflective narrative
Assessment done on admission – often the initial care plan sets the pattern of care without continuous assessment and evaluation	Assessment or pattern appraisal of person's needs is a continuous process in which person's needs are constantly interpreted, negotiated and evaluated
Person reduced to a set of problems – both actual and potential	The whole person kept in focus as a background to identified specific needs
Problems tend to be diagnosed by practitioners	Problem identification a mutual process between persons and practitioners

BOX 4.5 (CONTINUED)

Nursing process	Reflective narrative
Evaluation tends to be descriptive	Progress notes are reflective as a continuous process of assessment, response and evaluation
Focus on physical aspects of care	Focus on holistic needs
Dificulty in setting appropriate plan and goals for for psycho-social and emotional needs reflecting their marginality to care	Psycho-social and emotional needs are integral focus of care
Mindset that something always needs to be written irrespective of value, most often written at end of shift	The practitioner only writes what is meaningful sand pragmatic as an on-going process to reflect care
Nursing process is disjointed, often poorly written, and inadequate representation of care to follow	Narrative is easy to read and complete as an unfolding journey of the person's experience as basis for continuation of care
Culture of oral tradition as primary form of communication reduces significance of care plan	Reflective narrative culture is primary form of communication supported by reflective handovers
Nurses do not think in terms of the nursing process	Narrative reflects a natural way to think about care
Practitioners pay lip service to care planning as they know it is not a meaningful or practical approach to care – leads to disengagement with the patient	Practitioners engrossed in reflective narrative as it also represents their own journey with the person – leads to engagement with the person

SUMMARY

How holistic practice is communicated from written and verbal contexts, formally and informally is the beating pulse of holistic practice. In Chapter 5 I explore how the delivery of holistic practice can be most effectively organised.

NOTES

1 The idea of 'smooth running' stems from Friedson's notion that the first and foremost goal of the organisation is its own smooth running (rather than patient care unless of course patient care becomes a problem and disturbs smooth running).See Friedson E (1970) *Professional dominance*. Aldine Atherton, Chicago.

2 These references are merely representative of the literature on patient involvement in decision making published in the 1990s.

3 Clearly. With the advent of computer records, storing notes at the foot of the bed is obsolete. However, holistic practitioners inform persons they can view their computer record or be informed 'this is what I have recorded about our dialogue.

4 There is a welter of information about written communication available on Google.

5 See Chapter 7 – System for living and ensuring quality.

REFERENCES

Ashworth P, Longmate M, and Morrison P (1992) Patient participation: its meaning and significance in the context of caring. Journal of Advanced Nursing 17; 1430–9.

Batehup L and Evans A (1992) A new strategy. Nursing Times 88(47); 40–1.

Belenkey M F, Clinchy B M, Goldberger N R, and Tarule J M (1986) *Women's ways of knowing: the development of self, voice and mind*. Basic Books, New York.

Biley F (1992) Some determinants that affect patient participation in decision making about nursing care. Journal of Advanced Nursing 17; 414–21.

Burnard P and Morrison P (1991) Nurses' interpersonal skills: a study of nurses' perceptions. Nurse Education Today 11; 1167–74.

Dawson J (1987) Evaluation of a community based night sitter service. In *Research in the nursing care of the elderly* (Ed. P Fielding) Wiley, Chichester p87–106.

De la Cuesta C (1983) The nursing process: from development to implementation. Journal of Advanced Nursing 8; 365–71.

Heron J (1975) *Six-category intervention analysis*. Human Potential Resource Group, University of Surrey, Guildford.

Howse E and Bailey J (1992) Resistance to documentation – a nursing research issue. Journal of Nursing Studies 29(4); 371–80.

Isaacs W (1993) *Taking flight: dialogue, collective thinking, and organized learning*. Centre for Organizational Learning's dialogue project. MIT, Massachusetts.

Johns C (1989a) To whom it may concern? Nursing Times 85(39); 60–1.

Johns C (1989b) *The impact of introducing primary nursing on the culture of a community hospital*. Master of Nursing dissertation, University of Wales, Cardiff.

Johns C (2022a) Engaging the reflective spiral: the second dialogical movement. In *Becoming a reflective practitioner* (sixth edition) (Ed. C Johns) Wiley Blackwell, Oxford p36–51.

Johns C (2022b) The learning organization exemplified by the Burford NDU model. In *Becoming a reflective practitioner* (sixth edition) (Ed. C Johns) Wiley Blackwell, Oxford p215–32.

Latimer J (1990) The nursing process re-examined: enrolment and translation. Journal of Advanced Nursing 22; 213–20.

Macleod M (1994) 'It's the little things that count': the hidden complexity of everyday clinical nursing practice. Journal of Clinical Nursing 3(6); 361–8.

McElroy A, Corben V, and McLeish K (1995) Developing care plan documentation: an action research project. Journal of Nursing Management 3; 193–9.

Paterson J G and Zderad L T (1988) *Humanistic nursing*. National league for Nursing, New York.

Rowe M and Perry M (1984) Don't sit down nurse it's time for report. Nursing Times 85(26); 42–3.

Street A (1991) *Inside nursing: a critical ethnography of clinical nursing*. State University of New York Press, Albany.

Trnobanski P (1994) Nurse-patient negotiation: assumption or reality? Journal of Advanced Nursing 19; 733–7.

Ward K (1988) Not just the patient in bed three. Nursing Times 84(78); 39–40.

Waterworth K and Luker K (1990) Reluctant collaborators: do patient swant to be involved in decisions concerning care? Journal of Advanced Nursing 15; 971–6.

White A (1995) The nursing process: a constraint on expert practice. Journal of Nursing Management 1; 245–52.

System for Organising Delivery of Holistic Practice

CHAPTER 5

Christopher Johns

Any practice implementing a vision of holistic practice must necessarily consider the most effective system to organise its delivery. At Burford we utilised primary nursing, which *probably* best facilitates holistic practice compared with other methods (see Table 5.1). I emphasise *probably* because in my experience primary nursing requires a supportive internal environment of practice due to its impact on practitioners. The legacy of primary nursing is 'the named nurse'[1] although this is often no more than lip service to individualised care.

With primary nursing, each patient and family is allocated a primary nurse who has responsibility for working with the person towards enabling the person to plan and meet their health needs. The primary nurse is accountable for all aspects of the patient's care. When the primary nurse is not 'on duty' a team of associate nurses continue the planned care although with license to change the person's plan as appropriate.

THE THERAPEUTIC TEAM

The therapeutic team is the *essential* internal environment of practice to support all systems for delivering holistic practice. As the Burford vision (Table 1.1) states –

> *The therapeutic team is a team where practitioners are available to each other in ways that mirror practitioners being available to patients.*

As such, there is reciprocity between the way practitioners are available to persons and the way practitioners are available to each other. Manthey (1980) highlights the significance of the therapeutic team from a primary nursing perspective –

> *In primary nursing, the ability of each nurse to deal openly and honestly with others, especially in problem situations, is absolutely essential and must be emphasised from the start.*

Practising within an effective therapeutic team, practitioners are mutually available to support and *lift* each other to higher levels of energy and practice.[2] The therapeutic team is a *collective poise* greater than the sum of practitioner's individual poise (see Chapter 1). Thus practitioners will be more available to each other for mutual support the greater their individual poise.

Holistic Practice in Healthcare: The Burford NDU Person-centred Model, Second Edition. Edited by Christopher Johns.

Table 5.1 Ways of organising delivery of patient care

Task allocation	Patient allocation	Team nursing	Primary nursing
Patient reduced to a set of tasks allocated on a daily basis to practitioners	Patients allocated to a practitioner on a daily basis	Splitting the unit into teams	Patient allocated to a primary nurse on admission with total responsibility, autonomy for the patient's total stay
Diffuse responsibility, limited autonomy, and fragmentation of relationship with patient	Increased responsibility for the person's total care (although some tasks such as doctor's rounds and medication often excluded as the domain of the unit leader). Increased potential for developing relationship with the patient	Resulting in more tasks to fewer patients [as task allocation] OR Patient allocation within the team	Enabling development of relationship. Works with associate nurses to ensure continuity of care in absence

Failure to establish the therapeutic team results in an unhealthy working environment that inevitably reduces the practitioner's ability to be available to persons. Without doubt, the holistic practitioner is vulnerable to situations for whatever reason, such as coping with a heavy workload, emotional entanglement, self-doubt, and unresolved conflict. However, the therapeutic team may not reflect normal pattern of relationships within nursing teams and within the wider multi-disciplinary team. As such, it needs to be cultivated. *This is a prime role of holistic leadership.* The first step is to acknowledge the essential nature of the therapeutic team and to explicitly set out its expectations and responsibilities of roles whereby all practitioners (primary and associate nurses, care assistants and ancillary staff):

- 'Sign up' to actively engage in creating and sustaining the therapeutic team.
- Respect and value each other's respective roles.
- Are concerned for and available to each other at all times (recognising that work can be stressful at times for whatever reason).
- Work collaboratively to deliver planned care to patients to ensure they receive a consistent and congruent care.
- Give and receive open and honest feedback to each other (without defensive behaviour) whenever necessary to ensure holistic practice.
- Respond to situations of conflict openly and collaboratively (rather than defensively) with the intention to learn through it (where every conflict situation is a potential learning opportunity within the dynamic learning culture).[3]

Support for the ideal of the therapeutic team is found in the words of the then UKCC code of conduct paper (1992)[4] that highlighted the significance of collaboration with regards to relationships within health care teams.

> *Each nurse should work in a collaborative manner with other health care professionals and recognize and respect their particular contributions within the health care team. Experience has demonstrated*

that such co-operation and collaboration is not always achieved if individual members of the team have their own specific and separate objectives and one member of the team seeks to adopt a dominant role to the exclusion of the opinions, knowledge and skill of its team members.

These words note that realising a collaborative team may be difficult due to contradictory behaviours within the team. It exposes the gap between the ideal and prevailing reality. Yet it is important to visualise this gap as the first step towards bridging it.

As Wheatley (1999:130) writes

Behaviours don't change just by announcing new values. We move only gradually into being able to act congruently with those values. To do this we have to develop much greater awareness of how we're acting; we have to become far more reflective than normal. And we have to help one another when we slip back into old behaviours – that is unavoidable – but when that happens, we agree to counsel one another with a generous spirit. Little by little, tested by events and crises, we learn how to enact these new values. We develop different patterns of behaviours. We slowly become who we said we wanted to be.

One particular type of 'old behaviour' that constrains realising the therapeutic team is the harmonious team (Johns 1992).

THE BARRIER OF THE HARMONIOUS TEAM

The harmonious team is essentially defensive to protect practitioners from anxiety reflected in such quotes as 'people in glasshouses do not throw stones', 'let sleeping dogs lie' or 'don't stir up a hornet's nest'. The rule is to maintain a façade of harmony. If the rule is broken then the person breaking the rule is seen as the problem rather than the underlying issue the person has raised. The existence of the harmonious team is evident in experiences that Gill shared in guided reflection.[5] In session 5 Gill shared an experience where she had avoided giving the night associate nurse feedback about the negative way this nurse had talked about a patient being heavy in his presence during handover. Gill expressed a concern about not upsetting people. She said, 'I go along with people and try not to put their noses out of joint.' She felt she should give the nurse feedback but did not know how to do it in a way that would minimise the nurse's discomfort. Gill said 'I felt very angry about this' and recognised the night nurse probably got the non-verbal message because the rest of the handover felt uncomfortable. Gill's difficulty in giving staff uncomfortable feedback was further demonstrated in a catalogue of experiences concerning working with a care assistant whose behaviour reflected an intolerant attitude towards 'difficult' patients. Gill recognised in supervision how angry she was at herself for not confronting the care assistant and the impact of not giving feedback was to undermine her relationship with this care assistant and damage her self-esteem.

Gill's experiences explicitly reveal the harmonious team as a barrier to giving and receiving feedback essential to the therapeutic team and its consequences for practitioners on their relationships, feelings and self-esteem.

To move from a harmonious team to a therapeutic team is a significant culture shift (see Table 5.2).

Table 5.2 The tension between the therapeutic team and the harmonious team

Harmonious team	Therapeutic team
Is concerned with maintaining a façade of togetherness or teamwork. It does not talk about difficult feelings between its members and seeks to protect its members from outside threat. Conflict is brushed under the carpet or is inadequately dealt with within the greater need to 'get on with people' – creating a façade of harmony where practitioners are not available to each other and where conflict is never resolved and festers leading to anxiety, stress, resentment, bullying that ultimately impacts on quality of care.	Where practitioners are available to each to work collaboratively to realise their shared vision, open to give and receive feedback, give mutual support at all times, and deal collaboratively and positively to resolve conflict.
Culture shift --→	

OWNERSHIP

A particular barrier to realising the therapeutic team in primary nursing is 'ownership'. Pearson (1988) acknowledged what he termed 'a new imperialism of primary nurses in ownership of their patients, replacing the old imperialism of patients being owned by doctors' (cited in Johns 1992:89).

In the 'pilot' case study with Gill many of her shared experiences concerned her relationship with the two primary nurses. Despite the hospital's vision's focus on collegial relationships within the therapeutic team, it was not being role-modelled in her day-to-day relationships. For example, in session 3 Gill reflected on her feelings concerning a patient whom she had admitted and who had been very upset. Ann, the primary nurse, had returned after 'days off' and 'took over' this patient's care, Gill commented 'I felt a little pushed out. I couldn't go up and continue my role with the patient. I felt a bit excluded. I felt a bit excluded. It was the same with T and M, it's difficult not to have anything to do with him today. If I had got involved Ann may have thought 'I was not looking after the patients I had today.'

In session 13 Gill related an incident where Tina had been in the office when a relative of one of the patients asked to speak to her. Tina interjected, saying she was the primary nurse, and took over the conversation, leaving Gill 'feeling slighted in public'.

As she noted, 'Previously, because I was the one in charge of a shift I am the one the patients and relatives come to and it's quite difficult.' The lack of being acknowledged reinforced that patients belonged to the primary nurses and that associate nurses had a secondary role. Neither of the primary nurses recognised this problem and the frustration it caused Gill. Gill lacked the assertiveness to give the primary nurses feedback about how she felt despite working through these experiences in guided reflection. These incidents (amongst many others) exposed a lack of awareness and sensitivity both primary nurses had for the contribution Gill and other members of staff made to the care of 'their' patients that typified 'ownership' behaviour and its demoralising impact on those staff. Gill's difficulty accepting what she perceived to be a 'minor role' became evident when she reflected on her past experiences as a senior staff nurse.

Tina could sensitively let Gill continue her relationship with the person and family from a mentoring perspective, enabling Gill to gain confidence and expertise in becoming a primary nurse.

Table 5.3 Dilemmas between primary and associate nurses.

Primary nurses	
'I should involve associate nurses in care.'	'I must protect myself from interference.'
'I need help to make decisions about care.'	'I must protect myself from lack of experience (and competence).'
Associate nurses	
'Primary nurses should involve us in care.' 'My experience is now not acknowledged.'	'We must not step on their toes.'

A study of the impact of implementing primary nursing in another community hospital (Johns 1989) reinforced Pearson's observation in the way it had disrupted the 'normal' team. As one primary nurse commented, 'when I deliberately change something on the care plan I come back from my days off and it hasn't been carried out. Is it because they disagree with what's been written or are they too busy to read the care plan?' I could feel her frustration. Other nurses countered this comment by saying they resented less experienced nurses telling them what to do or that they had read the care plan and disagreed with it and had therefore disregarded it.

Another nurse noted, 'we went from being quite a good team where we used to work well together to people tending to go very much off on their own.'

It concluded that primary nursing had split the old team into two camps – 'then and us' characterised with interpersonal dilemmas towards the other group (see Table 5.3).

Clearly, it is essential for practice units to appreciate the potential barriers of the harmonious team whatever the system for delivering holistic practice is established and ownership if choosing to implement primary nursing as within the Burford NDU model. However, implementing primary nursing is not an imperative. The practice unit will need to weigh up whether it will help facilitate holistic practice challenging whether the current system is adequate and mindful of the significance of developing the therapeutic team.

STRESS AND BURNOUT

The therapeutic team is one safety valve for practitioners to release anxiety and stress rather than take it home and stew in it. All practice is potentially stressful no matter what system is utilised to organise the delivery of holistic practice yet perhaps more so with primary nursing.

An analysis of 52 experiences shared by Gill in her role as an associate nurse in the 'pilot' guided reflection case study revealed that 39 experiences were 'stressful' broken down as follows:

Workload	1
Being exposed as not competent	6
Interpersonal conflict	22
Working with 'difficult' patients	6
Working with doctors	3

As Gill's experiences indicate, situations of conflict were stressful, pulling away at her self-esteem, especially when conflict remains unresolved leaving behind a sense of unease. Conflict can be viewed on three levels:

Level 1– intrapersonal conflict within the practitioner

Level 2 – interpersonal conflict between the practitioner and the person/family

Level 3 – interpersonal conflict between the practitioner and colleagues and wider health-care team.

Gill experienced intrapersonal conflict as

- Fear of being seen as incompetent, which resulted in not seeking feedback as if feedback would expose her incompetence.
- Tension between old values and expectations from her role at Burford notably issues of control and professional involvement.
- Lack of poise in coping with emotional fall-out from situations of conflict with.
- Colleagues and with patients.

As Gill evidenced, her felt lack of support from her colleagues meant that these issues of conflict were not easily resolved and indeed added to her stress. People are not robots despite the effort to develop poise. Within an effective therapeutic team Gill's colleagues would have picked up her stress cues and supported her with its ethos of mutual support and mandate to deal openly and positively with situations of conflict. The therapeutic team views all conflict as a learning opportunity because it always points the way to some aspect of practice that is problematic. Wrapped up in intrapersonal conflict and self-concern with depleted energy the practitioner cannot be fully available to persons.

INTERPERSONAL CONFLICT

By far the most significant source of Gill's stress was interpersonal conflict with her colleagues because she did not feel acknowledged or supported by the primary nurses and felt powerless to confront this state of affairs despite exploring these issues within guided reflection. Understanding Gill's plight highlighted the vital work of developing the therapeutic team.

The stressed professional naturally seeks to protect self rather than be open to possibilities and learning new, more congruent ways of coping, to practice holistically. However, if stress is not dealt with adequately it inexorably leads to burnout – a descent into a black hole where the bonds that contain the self-snap. However, stress and burnout can be positively viewed as a healing space whereby the practitioner is allowed to descend into herself and as necessary to resolve stress and its causes. It may be dark, lonely and painful but it is still a healing space. Such healing is a journey of discovery not recovery because recovery suggests returning to what she was before – a self not coping, hurt, only for the self to be battered again. Hence the therapeutic team is the vital antidote to stress of everyday holistic practice. And yet, it must be actively cultivated.

SUMMARY

To reiterate, although primary nursing is not essential towards realising holistic practice it is best suited given the understanding of developing a genuine therapeutic team. No doubt, many practitioners would claim to be available to each other for support as necessary but evidence suggests that this is not the case within the pervasive harmonious team. As notes from Gill's guided reflection indicate, guided reflection is a space in which she could explore her experiences to gain insight towards becoming an effective holistic practitioner. This is the focus of Chapter 6.

NOTES

1 Turner noted – The named nurse concept stresses the importance of individualised care for patients. The concept is compatible with methods of nursing that put emphasis on the individual relationship with patients, such as primary nursing and team nursing. With sufficient resources, the named nurse is a suitable concept to apply in the organisation of care delivery in mental health nursing.

Turner H (1997) Incorporating the named nurse concept into care. *Professional Nurse* 12(8):582–584.

2 See chapter 1 regards lifting energy as a quality of holistic practice.

3 I utilise the Thomas and Kilmann conflict management model to help practitioners view and resolve conflict. The model sets out 5 modes of managing conflict: avoidance, accommodation, compromise, competition and collaboration. From the perspective of the therapeutic team collaborative modes need to be developed. Through reflection, the practitioner can position themselves within the five modes and then plot over time towards shifting to a collaborative mode. This is not necessarily easy to accomplish as research has shown that most nurses and managers use avoidance and accommodation in managing conflict.

See Cavanagh S (1991). The conflict management style of staff nurses and nurse managers. *Journal of Advanced Nursing*, 16; 1254–60.

Johns C (1992). Ownership and the harmonious team: barriers to developing the therapeutic team in primary nursing. *Journal of Clinical Nursing*, 1; 89–94.

Johns C (2022). *Becoming a reflective practitioner (sixth edition)* Wiley Blackwell, Oxford. (See figure 17.1, pages 190–1).Thomas K and Kilmann R (1974).

Thomas Kilmann conflict mode instrument. Xicom, Toledo.

4 The UKCC code of professional conduct was replaced by the NMC Code:

Professional standards of practice and behaviour for nurses, midwives and nursing associates (2021) (www.nmc.org.uk)

5 Gill was appointed as an associate nurse on the condition she entered into guided reflection with myself. The case study was a 'pilot' for introducing guided reflection with other practitioners. Hence Gill's reflections expose the existing hospital culture and its impact on herself. At this time, it is pertinent to note that the two primary nurses were in position prior to my arrival at the hospital and neither were as yet in guided reflection.Johns C (1992). 'Becoming a primary nurse: the first case study – a collaborative research case study to determine significant experiences for a nurse becoming a primary nurse at a Community Hospital (second edition)'. Unpublished research study University of Bedfordshire.

REFERENCES

Johns C (1989) *The impact of introducing primary nursing on the culture of a community hospital.* Master of Nursing Dissertation, University of Wales, Cardiff.

Johns C (1992) Ownership and the harmonious team: barriers to developing the therapeutic team in primary nursing. *Journal of Clinical Nursing* 1; 89–94.

Manthey M (1980) *The practice of primary nursing.* Blackwell Scientific Publications, Boston.

Pearson A (1988) *Primary nursing in the Burford and Oxford nursing development units.* Croom Helm, Sydney.

UKCC (1992) *Code of professional conduct* (third edition) London.

Wheatley M (1999) *Leadership and the new science. Discovering order in a chaotic world.* Berrett-Koehler publishers, San Francisco.

A System for Enabling Practitioners to Realise Holistic Practice

CHAPTER 6

Christopher Johns

In the previous chapter I noted Gill's experience in guided reflection. Guided reflection[1] was developed at Burford as the system towards enabling practitioners to realise holistic practice. It is a space where practitioners can reflect on and learn through their everyday experiences with a guide (and peers in group sessions) through focusing on and dialoguing to resolve the contradictions between realising holistic practice and the way they actually practice as recalled leading to insights to influence subsequent practice.

Through dialogue, the practitioner seeks to be in the 'right place' to be a holistic practitioner. As Mayeroff (1971:69) notes 'I am in place because of the way I relate to others. And place must be continually renewed and reaffirmed'. Being in the right place can never be taken for granted but a continuous developmental process.

Reflection on experience is most often triggered by some emotion or feeling that most often points towards an underlying contradiction or conflict although every experience is a potential learning opportunity. The type of experiences practitioners most reflect on relate to what Schon (1987) describes as the 'swampy lowlands' – those complex and indeterminate aspects of everyday practice wherein lie the greatest problems facing practitioners that are not easily solved by resorting to abstract theory (what Schön terms the 'hard high ground') due to their particular contextual and human nature. The guide feeds in relevant 'high ground' theory to inform and help frame and develop specific aspects of practice.

Undoubtedly, many aspects of holistic practice cannot be learnt from a theoretical perspective but only *meaningfully* through reflection on experience because of their contextual and subjective nature informed by relevant extant knowledge. These aspects include development of self and poise, ethics, attitude, reflection itself, communicative competence, responsibility, clinical judgement, perception.[2]

Through reflection on their experiences, practitioners naturally become increasingly reflective within practice itself, more attentive, more mindful of responding holistically to whatever is unfolding, where every experience is viewed as unique, as never having been experienced before, even though they may have experienced similar events before. As Paramananda (2001:138–9) informs –

> *Awareness sees everything as unique. Awareness brings an understanding that even the most common sight is never to be repeated and that to see something as it really is, we must be free from the habitual tendency to label and categorize. Only then can practitioners truly recognize things for what they are.*

Holistic Practice in Healthcare: The Burford NDU Person-centred Model, Second Edition. Edited by Christopher Johns.

STRUCTURED REFLECTION

Practitioners are encouraged to keep reflective journals to record and reflect on experiences that can later be shared and further reflected-on in guided reflection. Reflection is guided by using the Model for Structured Reflection [MSR]. The model was originally constructed from analysing pattern of dialogue from recorded guided reflection sessions (Johns 1998). The MSR is pragmatic, guiding the practitioner to explore the depth and breadth of experience towards gaining insight. It is a reflexive process of self-inquiry moving through seven dynamic interrelated stages moving from reflection in a journal to sharing and learning through guidance (Table 6.1). The 18th edition of the MSR is shown in Appendix 3.

GUIDANCE

Without doubt, skilled and continual guidance is vital to enhance the practitioner's learning through reflection. Meeting every 2–3 weeks for an hour with a practitioner would be ideal yet the reality of everyday practice may impinge.[3]

My initial approach to guidance is straightforward. Face to face with a practitioner I ask 'tell me your story' in much the same way the practitioner will establish a relationship with a person. Hence there is synchronicity between holistic care and holistic learning.

Table 6.1 Stages of reflection

Stage	
Preparatory	Bringing the mind home or clearing the head of distractions to bring oneself fully available to reflect. Learning this ability is an essential aspect of holistic practice of bringing oneself fully present to a person (as noted in the Being Available Template – Table 1.1).
Descriptive	Recalling and recording an experience in a journal paying attention to detail. As a consequence, the practitioner learns to pay attention to all aspects of practice in practice, or put another way to gain a holistic perspective.
Reflective	Using a series of cues [MSR] to explore the experience to draw out significance and contradiction towards understanding and realising holistic practice. Over time, the practitioner absorbs these cues as a natural way of thinking in practice itself to become a reflective practitioner essential to holistic practice.
Anticipatory	Imagining experiencing a similar situation to explore other creative ways of responding and their consequences and barriers. In doing so, the practitioner opens their mind to exploring new ways of thinking, perceiving and responding, challenging previous horizons of possibility.
Insightful	Drawing tentative insights from reflection to reflexively inform future practice.
Deepening insights	This has two interlocking aspects: 1. Dialogue between one's tentative insights with relevant extant theory. 2. Dialogue with guides in guided reflection to draw, challenge and deepen insights.
Debriefing and summarising	Debrief between the practitioner and guide to debrief and summarise learning to reflexively pick up during next guided reflection session.
Representation	Summarising and communicating insights in journal – to pick-up at the next session and for keeping a professional portfolio indispensable for demonstrating professional development.

The guide challenges and supports the practitioner to perceive and understand things for what they really are and to explore how the practitioner could respond differently, more in tune with their holistic beliefs. In doing so, the guide challenges the practitioner's partial perspectives and offers wider perspectives for the practitioner to consider and those barriers that might constrain the practitioner such as issues as necessary holistic skills and knowledge, one's attitude, and liberating self from aspects of previous ways of acting that had become embodied as noted in Chapter 2.

Advantages of being the guide and leader:

- It enables the leader to actualise their leadership role by being 'of service' to the practitioner towards enabling them to develop and realise holistic practice.
- It enables the leader to role model dialogue and work towards establishing collaborative relationships with practitioners that naturally spill over into everyday practice.
- It enables the leader to get direct feedback as to practitioner's competence and quality of care. Hence the leader feels in touch with their finger on the quality button alongside other measures.[4]
- It enables the leader and practitioner to tackle issues together as appropriate.
- It enables the leader to reflect on and learn through the experience of guiding the practitioner leading to a greater appreciation of holistic practice and holistic leadership.

The guide is mindful of creating a safe environment for the practitioner to disclose experiences. Key to this is the practitioner setting the agenda over what to share, the guide being non-judgemental and being mindful of giving advice (unless specifically asked for – 'what would you do in the situation?'), mutual disclosure (I would share my own experiences), confidentiality (this is between you and me).

If the practitioner felt that the guide is pursuing their own agenda by using guided reflection as a supervisory tool, then trust between the guide and practitioner would breakdown and the value of guided reflection diminished. The relationship would become guarded rather than open – a contradiction with holistic practice.

The practitioner may avoid sharing certain experiences that involve the leader because of learnt subordinate behaviour. The leader aware that such experiences are not being shared, can guide the practitioner to put their 'working relationship' into focus thus breaking down previous learnt hierarchical behaviour.

Yet it can be tricky for the guide to find the balance between being facilitative and directive in guiding the practitioner notably with practitioners who are inexperienced, set in their ways, or lack commitment towards realising holistic practice. Guidance then may feel like 'pulling teeth'. In response the guide may lose patience and become more directive in their anxiety to realise holistic practice (Johns 1988). Clearly, the guide needs to be mindful of any intolerance towards the practitioner, mindful of not labelling the practitioner as 'difficult'. Thus an attitude of 'positive regard' is vital to nurture whereby the guide believes the practitioner has the undoubted potential to develop. Where the guide feels intolerant for whatever reason, then this must necessarily be a focus to explore and resolve. As I noted in my doctoral thesis (Johns 1988; 312)

I was conscious of labelling Myrna as 'not having the right norms', even though I knew her difficulties when I appointed her as a primary nurse. I had planned to support her and yet it took seven sessions before I was able to feel positive towards her. I noted in my diary 'very conscious of my generally negative vibes towards

Myrna – I believe these stem from my perceptions of her suitability to be my image of a primary nurse'. I could hear my irritation with her during our early sessions but when I was eventually able to discuss these feelings with her, she said she had not perceived this. When I fed-back (in session 8) my perception of her compulsive tidying, her rigidity, her unpredictable moods, all within the need to control her environment, she said 'I fear being seen as incompetent for caring for people physically – I have been socialised into that.

I sensed Myrna's profound discomfort 'Is it uncomfortable to talk with me like this?'

Myrna replied 'I'm feeling quite tearful at the moment.'

I replied 'Because I might see you as incompetent?'

Myrna had difficulty in responding 'This is important – to be seen as competent but not in traditional nursing eyes but competent in new ways.'

This was an important turning point in our relationship. I wrote in my diary – 'I feel a wave of compassion in reading how I confronted Myrna with her compulsive behaviour in order to control her environment.'

It was a very intimate and emotional moment, and converted my residual irritation towards her into 'positive regard'. Myrna let go of her need to control and it marked the beginning of her real involvement in guided reflection that paralleled her real involvement with her patients. Perhaps this was the right time to act. Perhaps confronting her earlier may have been too destructive.'

Guidance can be viewed along a continuum depending on the practitioner's situation (Table 6.2).

Table 6.2 A developmental approach to guided reflection

Providing a facilitative response to the practitioner's increasing awareness of both the utility and limitations of their feelings and actions- reflecting the practitioner's growth to continuously monitor themselves and recognising the centrality of themselves to the effective realisation of holistic practice within the therapeutic team
Balance of high challenge and high support
Providing authoritative and definitive solutions and advice to the practitioner including the application of extant knowledge in response to presenting contradictions between a vision of holistic practice and its lived reality with a primary focus on development of self in relationship with both guide and persons.
The practitioner reaches 'master level' characterised by personal autonomy, insightful awareness, personal security, stable motivation, and an awareness of the need to confront their any problems that interfere with realising holistic practice. (adapted from Stoltenberg and Delworth Developmental model 1987)

(Adapted from Ralph's Developmental milestones' 1980)

FRAMING INSIGHTS

Insights change practitioners in terms of attitude, perception, and behaviour. They widen and shift the practitioner's horizons of knowing and being. To guide the practitioner to draw insight a number of framing perspectives were developed.[5]

The Being Available Template (Table 1.1) offers practitioners a comprehensive framework to both know and monitor the development of their holistic practice given the centrality of 'being available' to holistic practice.

EXEMPLARS

Three exemplars recorded from dialogue with Burford practitioners[6] in guided reflection raise significant points about the nature of both guided reflection (the process) and holistic practice (the intended outcome).

Layer the 'Being available template' over the exemplars to note its significance and to draw your own insights and how these might impact on your own clinical judgement, leadership and teaching.

Exemplar1: Mrs. Banning[7]

Roger[8] is a primary nurse at Burford.

Roger: 'She was such a one off. You couldn't imagine anyone like her. Her GP said she was an obsessive, neurotic and anxious lady. When she arrived here there was a look of sheer terror on her face. I had to respond. She said "Dr Pressley promised me a single room". I responded "I might have one when it's free (but) that might be a long time of never. I don't know. You can have some privacy by drawing the curtains around you." She said that she couldn't possibly sleep on a bed, that she had to sleep upright in a chair with pillows to support her back. I arranged for this and told her that Dr Pressley had asked for her to elevate her legs. She accepted this and put them on a stool. She said she was in a lot of pain. I asked her where it was and when she last had painkillers. I offered her two co-proxamol at one with some cold water. She said she couldn't stand cold water and indicated to her flask of hot water.'

CJ: 'How did you feel when she said that?'

Roger: 'I momentarily felt put out but then I went along with the things she wanted in order to help relieve her anxiety. She also wanted a strong cup of coffee in her cup and saucer and some biscuits from her tin. I want to pour the coffee and she said "I can do that, I am not helpless."'

CJ: 'Did that make you feel clumsy?'

Roger: 'Yes, a bit, but I was happy to go along with whatever she wanted. I asked her about what she knew about her illness, why she was here and what support she had. She said she didn't want to talk about that now, so I went away.'

CJ: 'You interpreted that as a dismissal?'

Roger: 'Yes. It was 8 p.m. when she arrived – she was quiet, calm, and grateful. She called me matron – she called me that all the time she was here, never referred to me as Roger except one. She liked to be called Mrs. Banning. She was very firm about that.'

CJ: 'Did anyone ever call her by her Christian name?'

Roger: 'I think one person did but she didn't respond... reflecting on the consequences of my action, I felt I did help her reduce her anxiety. She was comfortable in her chair and she was surrounded by familiar objects – her biscuits, clothes, dressings etc. She had arranged these things around her bed, with all her crockery, cutlery, newspapers, and books on tables in front of her and at the side of her. The curtains were drawn to the right hand side of her bed to make a private space. What's interesting about the way she had arranged her bed space was that it just like a nest – during the time she was here she pulled the curtains back until they were fully opened and she seemed happy to be seen.'

CJ: 'Did you ask her what made her pull the curtains back?'

Roger: 'No but I checked out that she was happy here – I reflected on alternative actions – I could have ignored her to get on with the other patients or got her to lie on the bed and to follow our instructions or responded with irritation to her anxiety, following the GP's advice not to show her any sympathy. However, the consequences of these interventions is that she would probably remain ultra anxious. How did I feel when it was happening? I felt instinctively she was not unlikeable but her palpable tension made me feel concerned for her. I wanted badly to help her feel comfortable. How did the patient make me feel? She seemed to feel more calm and at ease. My assumption was made from her appearance and non-verbal communication. How did I know how she felt? She accepted my actions, she became quiet and noticeably unmasked her terror and pain, the way she arranged her bedside, her warmth towards me and Shelly [night associate nurse] on the handover walk-round, and how she became more openly warm in her responses to people, and her improved mobility – she could hardly walk or even stand on admission. Early one morning I noticed she had walked out to the single room to visit another patient. She didn't want to show the day staff she could walk! What have I learnt? That responding directly to an anxious person's agenda may lead to significant reduction in anxiety and allow the commencement of a therapeutic relationship.'

CJ: 'Did you feel you were rivals for control of the environment?'

Roger: 'In some ways definitely, but I felt it was more important she had control than I did. If I had tried to take control there is an even bigger risk that she would have discharged herself and no chance of a positive admission. When she came in I had the feeling she was going to go home and that this wasn't going to work.'

CJ: 'Were you able to give the GP feedback about his briefing for her coming into hospital?'

Roger: 'Yes, but he was sceptical about how it would endure after she had gone home. He had a very laidback attitude towards her.'

CJ: 'Well, he had written her off. I expect she knew that. How did your colleagues react to her?'

Roger: 'They found her difficult at times, and at other times had good relationships with her and responded warmly to her. Certain staff felt we indulged her far too much and we shouldn't allow patients to express and have their individual needs met to such an extent. These staff to some extent ignored the philosophy and the rational of the holistic model.'

CJ: 'Did that threaten to undo the trust you had established with Mrs. Banning?'

Roger: 'In fact Mrs. Banning threatened to report one of the care assistants. I felt more like an anthropologist than a nurse dealing with Mrs. Banning.'

COMMENTARY

Roger's experience with Mrs. Banning reveals his ability to tune into and flow with her. He was able to shrug off the GP's label of Mrs. Banning as difficult in order to see her as a suffering person. He illustrates his concern and ability to tune into Mrs. Banning's wavelength and shows poise in dealing with his own feelings. He exposes a practice culture where not everybody is fully on board with the holistic vision, especially care assistants who were more engrained with previous ways of working and less in tune with holistic values. As clinical leader guiding Roger, such information led me to raise issues at handover – 'How do we find Mrs. Banning?' enabling staff to voice their feelings. It also prompted me to convene monthly group-guided reflection with the care assistants where such experiences can be explored and attitudes shifted.

Roger illustrates his self-questioning using MSR cues. Indeed I had very little input into the session beyond posing some pertinent questions. Simply by telling and reflecting on this experience enabled Roger to think about and makes sense of his practice, honing his reflective and holistic skills.

An aspect of mindfulness is *Apramada* – 'mindful attention to guard against unskilful action' (Sangharakishita 1998:146–7). By unskilful action I mean concerns that interfere with the practitioner being available to the other. These concerns emerge through Roger's narrative, guiding him to gain insights about such concerns and develop his poise.

Exemplar 2: Hilda[9]

This second exemplar concerns Jade's experience with Hilda. Like Leslie, Jade is a primary nurse. She reflects on her experience with Hilda in her associate nurse role.

Jade: 'Hilda told me I was horrid. I asked her why? She said it was because I had made her stand and take a few steps. I reminded Hilda that she had agreed to this action with the primary nurse and her husband the previous day as recorded on the care plan. Her response to this was "I didn't agree to anything no matter what anyone said!" Hilda implied that "we enjoyed bullying her" which upset me. I told her "if we wanted things to be easy we would just leave you" which brought an almost predicable response from Hilda "just leave me alone", which I then did. I felt pressured at this time with the need of other patients. It made me feel uncomfortable all morning.'

CJ: 'Could you have responded differently to her?'

Jade: 'No, I don't think so... it would be just the same. I had taken the right decision and made the right action based on the chat I had with the primary nurse yesterday.'

CJ: 'You seem angry with Hilda?'

Jade: 'It puts me in a dilemma... we don't come to work dressed in a suit of armour to protect yourself from all this shit... you just feel you are a target for people to fire at. This experience has affected my relationship with Hilda. I went back later to do her dressing and she just pulled away from me, didn't communicate, closed her eyes to dismiss me.'

CJ: 'So now, on reflection... what sense do you make of this experience?'

Jade: 'The dilemma of whether I should have tried to make Hilda do as she had agreed against her wishes. I recognise I was pressured. What do you think?'

CJ: 'Well... as an associate nurse she should not blindly follow planned care. You need to make a judgement as to whether Hilda's planned care was still appropriate for her needs. Whether Hilda agreed to one thing yesterday is history. She may have merely complied yesterday and now, faced with the reality of her decision, she feels quite differently.'

Jade: 'That puts it into perspective... I need to swallow my anger and talk with her about how she is feeling. That will help me discharge this residual anger and guilt I feel.'

CJ: '"The maxim – turning negative energy into positive energy for taking action!" A few days later Jade asked if we could have another guided reflection session if I was available later that afternoon after her shift finished.'

Jade: 'I have continued to feel awful about this experience. I should have gone back to talk with her but it was so busy I let it slide. However I have rationalised it as my oversensitivity. I was unable to avoid these awful feelings because of my concern for Hilda. Her rejection of me made me feel angry. I blamed her when in fact my approach was wrong. I feel I am on a merry-go-round of energy sapping emotions towards myself and towards Hilda.'

CJ: '"Beating yourself up is not helping anyone?" As I read it, your dilemma is deciding what would be therapeutic for Hilda. On one hand Hilda hates being in hospital and wants to go home to be with her husband but, on the other hand, she wants to be left alone because she felt so tired. Hence she is ambivalent about her rehabilitation and her level of dependence on us.'

Jade: 'I hadn't read his pattern. It makes sense.'

CJ: 'I sense your guilt reflects the way you perceive yourself as failing to care. Dickson (1982) describes a "compassion trap" whereby practitioners get trapped by their own concern or ethic of care, as if they have assumed all responsibility for the way the patient feels.'

Jade: 'I had better read that book! I know I should have gone back to talk with Hilda about my problem rather than her problem... our communication broke down. I became the anxious parent belittling Hilda and she rejected this imposed child role. I can image a sub-text "don't talk to me like that young lady, I'm old enough to be your grandmother!" [Jade laughs breaking the tension] I was trying to control the situation and my anxiety linked to pressure of work.'

CJ: 'I'll hit you with another theory worth reading. Noddings (1984) noted the practitioners' sense of being overwhelmed, resulting in feelings of guilt and conflict, was the inescapable risk of caring. The balance between concern and poise to guard against being overwhelmed is a fine line. On another note, have you talked this experience over with your colleagues?'

Jade: 'No I haven't because I didn't want to burden them with my problems.'

CJ: 'Do you think you should? You'll not be surprised about how common this experience is for them as well. It's not healthy to "stew in your own juices and stoke self-harm,"[10] limiting the opportunity to take your armour off.'

Jade: 'It's not just that... I didn't want to admit to Leslie (the primary nurse) that I messed up.'

CJ: '"So how do you now extricate yourself from this emotional entanglement?" (Jade is silent) OK. Visualise a space between us to put these residual feelings so we can look at them objectively.'

Jade: 'OK... that's helpful. I can see now I lost my poise. I could have said to Hilda – "I can see you don't want to do that – can we talk about that" and the situation would have been resolved without loss of face for both of us. I can see how this is tuning into her wavelength and flowing with her as you've mentioned before and which I totally respect. Indeed I'll go and have a word with her now.'

CJ: 'You say – have a word with her... yet what is your aim?'
Jade: 'To make peace... umm... what is my aim?'
CJ: 'Think about your communication strategy using Heron's "Six-category intervention analysis[11]"?'
Jade: 'That's a useful idea. I'll work through his categories... Giving information "You need to walk to get home."Giving advice/confrontation "if you want to get home you need to walk to make it easier for your husband to care for you".Catharsis "You seem reluctant Hilda. Why is that?" Catalytic – "Let's talk Hilda about your resistance to walking." Support "I know this is tough for you especially when you feel tired. I'm here to support you." That's amazing how Heron's typology helps me develop communicative competence from an adult-adult perspective.'
CJ: 'Yes, it's most useful.What do you need to now do?'
Jade: 'Armed with these ideas go back to Hilda and write up a SI sheet.'
CJ: 'Consider talking it over with your colleagues?'
Jade: 'Yes, that's most important.'
CJ: 'Holistic practice is not necessarily easy?'
Jade: 'Yep, but I wouldn't have it any other way!'

COMMENTARY

In contrast with Roger's experience, Jade fails to tune into Hilda's wavelength. Instead she tries to force Hilda into her own wavelength as dictated by the care plan. Jade's experience reveals how situations can fluctuate presenting a dilemma as to how best to respond, as if competing with the Hilda for control of the situation resulting in Hilda's comment that Jade was horrid. Perhaps Jade is less concerned about Hilda because she is not her primary nurse – 'just following care'. Jade does not want to change the care plan although she knows she has the authority to do so. What had been agreed yesterday fell apart today.

Jade is reluctant to 'burden her colleagues', admitting she didn't want the primary nurse to think she had 'messed up' or felt 'guilty'. I challenged her on her responsibility to foster the 'therapeutic team' to challenge and support each other.

The idea of visualising a 'space' to put feelings into offered Jade the opportunity to look at her feelings of anger and guilt more objectively. In acknowledging and working through these feelings, they can be converted into positive feelings about self and Hilda where anger is transformed and guilt shredded.

Note how dialogue with extant theory was helpful to enable Jade to 'see her situation more clearly and possibilities for responding differently, more in tune with holistic practice.

At the end of each guided reflection session I ask the practitioner 'How do you now feel?' to enable them to wrap up the session (see Table 6.1) by 'mopping up' their feelings and summarising what 'actions' to take as a consequence. These 'actions' are seeds planted in her mind to draw on in future experiences. Jade hadn't managed to deal with her emotional fallout from the first session and asked for another session where she was able to work through her resultant feelings and explore her communication skills in response to Hilda.

Jade's experience illuminates that it is vital the guide acknowledges the practitioner's feelings and emotions as valid. It is an aspect of being human. Words by Blackwolf and Gina Jones's are inspiring – 'Reflect periodically throughout the day. See clearly who you are, what you are experiencing. Like brother eagle, preen your emotional feathers throughout the day. They are the feathers that help you fly to greater heights.' (1996:15).

Exemplar 3: Kate,[12] Mavis and Joy[13]

Being an associate nurse at Burford is Kate's first position since graduating as a registered nurse. As a condition of her employment she contracted guided reflection. We pick up her reflection in session 13 – indicating she had been at Burford approximately 30 weeks[14] when she reflects on her relationship with Mavis, a woman admitted for respite care, and with Joy her daughter. Mavis is her first primary nurse patient.

Session 13

Kate: 'It's the first time I've seen Mavis as Joy has described her at home. For the last few months Joy has been saying how demanding she's been, that she doesn't want Joy to go out. Joy's saying she feels trapped, that it is affecting her marriage. I haven't seen that before when Mavis was here. I'm just observing how she is this time. She is much more demanding, for example, "take off my tights", "put that there", and suchlike.'

CJ: 'What are your choices?'

Kate: 'To go along with it.'

CJ: 'Do you have other choices?'

Kate: 'To challenge Mavis's behaviour; for example, to ask her to be more polite, to ask her why she is acting differently than before.'

CJ: 'What would be the consequences of "going along with it"?'

Kate: 'She would receive care similar to what she gets at home.'

CJ: 'Is that significant?'

Kate: 'It is in terms of the respite care philosophy not to disrupt people's normal life style... and yet we also view respite care as enabling the carers to care more effectively and give emotional and psychological support.'

CJ: 'OK... so we may have a dilemma as to how best to respond. Does her daughter everything for at home?'

Kate: 'Yes.'

CJ: 'But grudgingly?'

Kate: 'Yes, I think it's getting that way.'

CJ: 'You're not sure?'

Kate: 'I'm not sure "grudgingly" is the right word. Joy is getting tired that's for sure.'

CJ: 'But Joy is complaining to you?'

Kate: 'She's justifying it; what Mavis did for her when she was a little girl.'

CJ: 'Like repaying debts... caring from a sense of duty?'

Kate: 'Yes very much.'

CJ: 'Are you doing something you don't want to do by mirroring Joy's behaviour with her mother at home?'

Kate: 'It's not something you want to do. I'm carrying on for Joy's sake.'

CJ: 'But you would like to change Mavis's behaviour to make Joy's life easier. Therefore why carry on?'

Kate: 'Because it's the only way to observe the full picture at the moment.'

CJ: 'Let's look at your options to challenge Mavis?'

Kate: 'If I challenged her she might act differently than she does at home.'

CJ: '"Are you thinking that you might succeed in changing her behaviour here in hospital but not at home?" Kate: "Yes, if I ask her to be polite in hospital when she's here, she would try desperately hard. Mavis is morally correct. It would upset her too much. She would look at me with wide-eyes wonder and disbelief."'

CJ: 'Would you be asking her to be polite for your benefit rather than hers?'
Kate: 'It wouldn't be for me. It would be for Joy's sake.'
CJ: 'What might be the reasons for her acting differently? Could the reasons possibly be organic or dementia?'
Kate: 'I'm not sure about that although it's important to put her behaviour into that perspective. It's definitely possible. I feel she is in a strop because Joy has gone on holiday. She didn't want Joy to leave her.'
CJ: 'This has been happening for two years now. Do you think she has become more dependent? Could you use a cathartic response to enable her to surface this anger – for example "you seem angry that Joy has gone on holiday"?'
Kate: 'Thinking about the cathartic and catalytic ways of responding[15] I don't think I often do that. That's why I probably chose to "carry on as before" strategy because I have a fear of using these types of responses. I haven't used them before.'
CJ: 'You probably have but not in such a deliberative way. Perhaps you are avoiding delving into Mavis's feelings because of fear – fear of the unknown? Fear of upsetting Mavis? Fear of cocking it up?'
Kate: 'Yes, upsetting Mavis... being confrontational. Mavis has some environmental problems being here. There's a nosey woman in the same room and sharing a room with a man as well. It can't be easy for her.'
CJ: 'Are you suggesting that Mavis may be angry with us for these reasons? Consider the Burford cue – "what factors are important for this person to make their stay in hospital comfortable".'
Kate: 'I hadn't considered whether these factors could have made her discontented.'
CJ: 'Something else for you to consider? Do you feel you have a good relationship with Joy?'
Kate: 'I feel she trusts me all of a sudden. I've always been open and friendly with her. I thought no more about it until I became her primary nurse. I don't know what else I need to do with her.'
CJ: 'That seems a significant insight. One idea might be to invite her for a chat when she returns from her holiday ostensibly to feedback how Mavis has been in hospital? How does that feel? (Kate nods...) How do you now feel about Mavis?'
Kate: 'I did think she was a very nice lady. Now, I'm beginning to think she is more manipulative than I gave her credit for.'
CJ: 'Does that make you feel?'
Kate: 'Hesitant.'
CJ: 'It's important for you to understand how you feel about her because it may influence your responses to her?'
Kate: 'That may be why I was going to observe her.'
CJ: 'How do you feel about Joy?'
Kate: 'I feel protective towards her, more protective towards her than I do about Mavis.'
CJ: 'Are you at risk of being caught between two people?'
Kate: 'Definitely... not knowing were my priorities lie.'

COMMENTARY

Kate's frustration triggers her reflection. The tension between holistic intent and actual practice vibrates through our dialogue. Observe the way Kate responds as the drama unfolds. It gives an impression that Kate expects the family to fit into her wavelength and yet over time

Kate shifts as she comes to understand Mavis and Joy's situated meaning and shifts to flow with them. Yet Mavis and Joy have different and potentially conflicting wavelengths, so Kate must find her way to move along both simultaneously.

In guided reflection it is imperative for the guide to be non-judgemental and patient – often talking around the topic as if every turn opens more light for the practitioner to see things more clearly. As the guide I am mindful of planting seeds in Kate's mind to germinate at a later time, perhaps in practice, on reflecting on our last session or at any time, perhaps in the middle of the night – a sense of 'eureka, I get it!'. And yet, in this session I was more directive in response to Kate's uncertainty and emotional entanglement we try to unravel the experience so Kate can see herself objectively as being entangled in the precarious family dynamics. Only then can she work at new ways of being to extricate herself yet remaining available to them.

Through the dialogue I metaphorically hold Kate's hand so she move more safely across this swampy lowland of her practice, perhaps to an extent pulling her out of the swamp she had slipped into.

Part of Kate's difficulty was a tension between conforming to some idea of how a nurse should respond and being authentic. Exploring her experience she could acknowledge her real self as worthy, legitimising and valuing her qualities of being open and honest. As Jourard (1971:184) noted

> ***People learn to squash their real selves because they have learned to fear the consequences of authentic being and blind themselves to much of their real self; impairing their ability to empathise with patients and disclose themselves.***

Clearly conforming to some stereotype of 'what a nurse should be' is not conducive to holistic practice. Of course, knowing your real self in order to be authentic is not easy or even desirable, for example not liking the other person. Do you then become a chameleon hiding your true colours?[16] As Yoko Beck (1989:92) notes 'If you had to define "true self", what would you say?'

Session 20

Kate continued to reflect on her relationship with Mavis and Joy through subsequent sessions linked to further respite care admissions. In session 20 Kate again shared her experience concerning with Mavis and Joy.

Kate: 'Mavis is now very confused and very sad. Joy says Mavis is more confused and that she doesn't know what to do about it, how to keep Mavis occupied. Mavis is less able to do her knitting, even to watch TV.'

CJ: 'And making more demands on Joy as a result?'

Kate: 'Joy feels she should be spending more time with Mavis whilst she is in here.'

CJ: 'Can you reassure Joy about that?'

Kate: 'I said that we will try and stimulate Mavis more whilst she is in hospital and pass on any tips to Joy and Wilf for them to try out at home.'

CJ: 'Has anything emerged?'

Kate: 'She can talk about the past with some understanding. Therefore old photographs or video would be useful.'

CJ: 'We have a book in the library on reminiscence (Coleman1986) that might be a useful reference for you to explore?'

Kate: 'Joy would have to sit with her to accomplish that. She won't go to any clubs because she's deaf. Yet she will sit with Ethel (another patient) and have a conversation. I really think she plays Joy up at home, I really do. I'm toying with the idea of a home visit to clarify in my own mind if that is so.'

CJ: 'Even if she was, what could you do about it?'

Kate: 'I'm not sure if I could do anything except be more empathic.'

CJ: 'How do you feel about this situation?'

Kate: 'Frustrated! I know I am absorbing some of Joy's anxiety, I know that, and I am trying hard not to, but it's difficult when you are involved with people like this... that's why it's so helpful to share it with you... not just get ideas or check out my own, but to help me keep things in perspective.'

CJ: 'That's so honest of you. OK, let's focus on other options. What about other workers, for example the Community Psychiatric nurse [CPN] for the elderly?'

Kate: 'No. The only contact is the GP. They have a lot of trust in him.'

CJ: 'Have you thought about the CPN as a resource?'

Kate: 'No, but that's a good idea. I haven't met her. This would be a good opportunity to do that.'

CJ: 'Do you know how to contact her? Her contact is in the resource file.'

Kate: 'Knowing the home situation would lead to a better appreciation of her life pattern and give me insight into the way Mavis and Joy normally relate to each other and the help Joy gives Mavis. For example, if Joy is helping Mavis to dress at home and Mavis was managing that for herself here, we could help Joy change her management for Mavis at home.'

CJ: 'Of course the dynamics are different at home – Mavis may be more dependent to get Joy to help her, and Joy may want to help more than we might because of her perceived dutiful daughter role. We've talked about this role and her guilt before. Again, the CPN may help you with a cognitive assessment of time/space/place orientation etcetera. Do you need to consider whether that would be appropriate or just intrusive? You feel hesitant about a home visit?'

Kate: 'I feel claustrophobic about Joy and Wilf. I feel almost smothered by their love. I'm dodging them! It makes me reluctant to go and to feel even more closed in by them... stupid things like them calling me "sweetheart"!'

CJ: 'I recall your aversion to being called names of endearment by Elizabeth [another patient]. You can't accept that from Joy and Wilf? Use the Transactional Analysis template to position yourself?[17]'

Kate: 'I have to be in a certain mood to accept it. I can see the TA pattern – parent/child with me resisting their loving parenting! I know I should be mindful to stay in adult mode, not to go into child mode. I appreciate this "up here" [in guided reflection] but it's different when I'm "down there" [in the ward].'

CJ: 'It feels like a situation of entanglement – of losing the boundaries between yourself and them. You are aware of this and now need to take a step back to untangle yourself and yet they want you to take a step forward.'

Kate: 'Yes, I'm trying to maintain a professional distance.'

CJ: 'I'm not sure about this idea of "professional distance" – it sounds like a barrier to retreat behind because you cannot manage your emotions. This is a repeating theme through your experiences – where to pitch your involvement with patients and families. Perhaps you want to take a step back because you don't know what's waiting for you?'

Kate: 'In light of past experiences I guess I should have seen this coming but it's like it creeps up and grabs you. I don't know what demands it's going to make on me but it feels uncomfortable.'

CJ: 'Do you know the best ways to resolve this dilemma; on one hand knowing your responsibility to help them and, on the other hand, wanting to flee from them?'

Kate: 'I know a solution – to do the home visit but to spell out to them that the visit is not a social visit.'

CJ: 'In other words to set the boundaries for the visit and for your own relationship with them.'

Kate: 'Yes.'

CJ: 'I agree with your actions. It enables you to be positive rather than defensive. In doing so you don't need to resist them but accept their need to be affectionate to you. It gives you some control and anxiety makes people need to be in control. Do you feel able to be open and honest with them as before?'

Kate: 'Being in control – that's important. I can relate this to my earlier work with them, the way they make me feel like a "big soft puppy". I think I can deal with it now.'

CJ: 'Do they have children?'

Kate: 'Joy has two children from a previous marriage – are you suggesting they might want to mother me?'

CJ: 'It's a possibility. Your work now is to be assertive and re-establish an adult-adult relationship as the basis of a "working with" relationship.'

COMMENTARY

Kate's involvement with Joy and Wilf has taken a paradoxical turn. Having worked hard to connect with them she now recoils from the unexpected consequences. Joy and Wilf wish to reciprocate Kate's care at an unacceptable level. Hence Kate resists this demand, feeling smothered by love and treated like a little girl with such endearments as 'sweetheart'. Yet Kate also feels guilty of her resistance. As a result she has again become entangled, trapped by her 'ethic of care' (Dickson 1982), caught in a dilemma of knowing how best to respond. She cannot reciprocate the level of involvement demanded by the family but neither can she resist it openly because of her concern for the family. In response to her anxiety, Kate has flipped into rebellious child mode fighting against 'her parents' who wished to impose a level of intimacy that was unacceptable and uncomfortable. Kate's work in guided reflection was to see herself entangled in a web of emotion and work towards unravelling herself to regain an adult-adult relationship and poise necessary to be available to Mavis and Joy. This is vital work for the holistic practitioners. As Kate noted she have had no preparation in her training for holistic practice. It is pertinent to ask what difference does holistic practice make to this family (or indeed to any person or family)? Couldn't Kate simply maintain her professional distance and not become involved in the family's dynamics and in doing so not open the can of worms? Or put another way – 'what is nursing?'

SUMMARY

Guided reflection is an effective developmental process to enable practitioners towards realising holistic practice as a lived reality. It also offers the guide as leader a meaningful way to fulfil a holistic leadership role. As the exemplars illustrate, guided reflection offers both practitioner and guide feedback about the nature of holistic practice and understanding and resolving contradictions faced by practitioners towards realising it as a lived reality as evident within the exemplars noted above and as noted in the previous chapter.

Guided reflection is also one way to live quality the focus of Chapter 7.

NOTES

1 My description of the nature of guided reflection is deliberately brief. The reader is referred to 'Becoming a reflective practitioner' [sixth edition] (Johns 2022) for in-depth exploration. Initially I termed guided reflection as 'professional supervision'. I changed it to 'guided reflection' because the word 'supervision' is traditionally concerned with controlling worker's performance.

See Johns C (1993) Professional supervision. *Journal of Nursing Management* 1(1); 9–18.

2 This understanding is significant in re-visioning the educational curriculum from a holistic and reflective perspective. See Johns C (2022) 'The Reflective curriculum'. In C.Johns (Ed.) *Becoming a reflective practitioner (sixth edition).* Wiley Blackwell, Oxford, pp. 151–166.

3 A time span of no less than 3 weeks is significant to ensure developmental continuity. However, personal development may be viewed as a lesser priority than patient care and postponed. Over 4 weeks, development looses continuity and momentum and becomes less effective and less valued (Johns 1998).

Johns C (1988) *'Becoming a reflective practitioner through guided reflection'*. Unpublished PhD thesis. The Open University, Milton Keynes.

4 I also worked two days a week on the 'shop floor' given direct care as an associate nurse so I was also getting feedback about the quality of care and ipso facto practitioner performance.

5 See Johns (2022) (op cit.) (Figure 5.2, page 55).

6 These exemplars were recorded as data in my doctoral research – see footnote 3.

7 A version of this narrative was previously published in *Becoming a Reflective Practitioner* [First edition] (2000: 85–87).

8 Roger Cowell is also author of the chapter 'Discovering the art of nursing: using the BNDU model at Burford' (chapter 9).

9 This text has been adapted from when it was first published in 1e of *Becoming a reflective practitioner* (2000:139–40).

10 I am quoting Lydia Hall – 'Anxiety over an extended period is stressful to all the organ functions. It prepares people to fight or flight. In our culture however, it is brutal to fight and cowardly to flee, so we stew in our own juices and cook up malfunction. This energy can be put to use in exploration of feeling through participation in the struggle to face and solve problems underlying the state of anxiety.'

Hall L (1964) Nursing – what is it? Canadian Nurse 60(2); 150–4. This quote captures the essence of guided reflection as an energy converter for taking positive action.

11 Heron J (1975) Six-category intervention analysis. Human Potential Resource Group, University of Surrey, Guildford.

12 Kate is also co-author with Jan Dewing of chapter – 'Just following care? Reflections of associate nurses in using the BNDU model at Burford'.

13 This text was published in *Becoming a reflective practitioner* 1e (2000: 144–61), and in 2e (2004:131–43).

14 Guided reflection sessions take place approximately every 3 weeks for one hour.

15 The notion of cathartic and catalytic interventions refers to Six-category intervention analysis (Heron 1975) – that offers a typology of communications skills that Kate had explored earlier in our guided reflection relationship – see footnote 5.

16 The tension between being authentic and being a chameleon is important to acknowledge. The tension inevitably emerges as the practitioner strives to become holistic. See Aranda S and Street A (1999) Being authentic and being a chameleon: nurse-patient interaction revisited. *Nursing Inquiry* 6;75–82.

17 Transactional analysis is a useful tool to enable practitioners to view themselves in relationship with others. The holistic practitioner seeks to construct and maintain adult-adult relationships with patients and families as the basis for 'working with' them. However for one reason or another, people slip into either parent or child modes, and in doing so exert pressure on the other to conform to a complimentary mode to ensure communication does not break down. Being mindful, Kate's work is to move into her necessary adult mode and enable Joy and Wilf to return to a complimentary adult role as the basis for their relationship. It sounds easy but as Kate demonstrates relationships can be difficult when one party exerts untenable expectations.

(See Stewart I and Joines V (2012) TA Today: a new introduction to transactional analysis. Russell Press, Nottingham).

REFERENCES

Aranda S K and Street A F (1999) Being authentic and being a chameleon: nurse-patient interaction revisited. *Nursing Inquiry* 6(2); 75–82.

Beck C Yoko (1989) *Everyday Zen.* Harper Collins, London.

Beck C Y (1997) *Everyday Zen.* Thorsons, London.

Blackwolf J and Jones G (1996) *Earth dance drum.* Commune-E-Key, Salt lake City.

Coleman P (1986) *Ageing and reminiscence processes: social and clinical applications.* Wiley Chichester.

Dickson A (1982) *A woman in your own right.* Quartet Books, London.

Hall L (1964) Nursing-what is it? *Canadian Nurse* 60(2); 150–4.

Heron J (1975) Six-category intervention analysis. Human Resource Research Project. University of Surrey, Guildford.

Johns C (1988) *Becoming a reflective practitioner through guided reflection.* Unpublished PhD thesis. The Open University, Milton Keynes.

Johns C (1998) *Becoming an effective practitioner through guided reflection.* Unpublished doctoral thesis. The Open University.

Johns C (2022) *Becoming a reflective practitioner* (sixth edition) Wiley Blackwell, Oxford.

Jourard S (1971) *The transparent self.* Van Nostrand, New York.

Mayeroff M (1971) *On caring.* Harper Perennial, New York.

Noddings N (1984) *Caring – a feminine approach to ethics and moral education.* University of California Press, Berkley.

Paramananda (2001) *A deeper beauty.* Windhorse, Birmingham.

Ralph N B (1980) Learning psychotherapy: a developmental perspective. *Psychiatry* 43; 243–250.

Sangharakshita (1988) *Know your mind: the psychological dimension of ethics in Buddhism.* Windhorse, Birmingham.

Schon D (1987) *Educating the reflective practitioner.* Jossey-Bass, San Francisco.

Stoltenberg C D and Delworth U (1987) *Supervising counsellors and therapists.* Jossey-Bass, San Francisco.

A System to Enable Practitioners to Live Quality

CHAPTER 7

Christopher Johns

In the previous chapter I set out guided reflection as a system to enable practitioners to become effective holistic practitioners. Ensuring quality is everybody's responsibility. Through dialogue both guide and practitioner gain feedback as to the quality of the practitioner's holistic practice. Through guided reflection practitioners become increasingly reflective within practice itself and in doing so 'live' quality.

Living quality has triple feedback loops:

1. Do practitioners realise holistic practice?
2. Is the vision of holistic practice appropriate?
3. How might holistic practice be improved?

These loops reflect the dynamic learning culture. Nothing is static. Everything is in dynamic movement.

The dynamic learning culture is reflected in clinical governance defined as

> *A framework through which Health Service organizations are accountable for continuously improving the quality of their services and safeguarding high standards of care by creating an environment in which clinical excellence will flourish. Clinical governance encompasses quality assurance, quality improvement and risk and incident management. (DHSS 1988/2022)*[1]

Quality is monitored externally in the UK through the Care Quality Commission (CQC). The CQC is a powerful stick to ensure organisations take quality seriously with its three pronged agenda of the patient's experience, patient safety, and clinical effectiveness. Yet the CQC visit is an external quality measure. Its approach is a blunt tool that views quality from a prescriptive lens, a broad snapshot that cannot capture the nuances of caring. Whilst all organisations must accept this external approach, it is not enough if practitioners accept responsibility to ensure quality of holistic practice. Organisations may have internal systems in place such as clinical audit, standard setting and clinical supervision. Burford hospital had previously utilised QUALPACS and Phaneuf's nursing audit, but these external measures were of dubious validity.[2] External measures are something imposed on the practice setting and may create a sense of passivity towards ensuring quality or even panic and false impression when a forthcoming CQC visit is announced.

Burford's approach to enable practitioners to 'live quality' was to develop 'Standards of care' and 'Clinical audit' as internal measures alongside guided reflection.

Holistic Practice in Healthcare: The Burford NDU Person-centred Model, Second Edition. Edited by Christopher Johns.

STANDARDS OF CARE[3]

Constructing standards of care is a process of team learning to enable practitioners to collectively reflect on discrete aspects of shared practice in order to develop its nature and quality thereby contributing to *creating an environment in which clinical excellence will flourish*. Standard setting is a creative process. Any aspect of practice, both clinical and organisational, can be the focus for a standard of care.

A standard of care is negotiated and agreed by all staff concerned in achieving its outcome. So for example, the cook and domestics would be involved on a standard about nutrition. GPs, homecare and district nurses, concerning a standard about discharge of patients. A standard can involve laypeople as representative of the wider community, for example Age Concern to review our standards as many of Burford's patients were elderly.

Standards of care reflect optimal quality – the tension between what is desirable and what is achievable. Clearly, standards need to be potentially achievable otherwise they are pipe dreams and create frustration. Yet standards also need to reflect desirability, as something to move towards.

STRUCTURE OF STANDARDS OF CARE

Standards are constructed around a standard statement and identifying relevant structure, process and outcome criteria that can be monitored [see Box 7.1].

BOX 7.1 STANDARDS OF CARE CRITERIA

Structure criteria	Process criteria	Outcome criteria
What resources are necessary to enable the standard to be achieved?	What actions do staff need to take to enable the standard to be achieved?	How might staff determine if the standard has been met?
These include	For example	For example
• Staff skills and attitudes skill mix • Number of single rooms • Maintenance contracts • Organisational policies • Equipment • Budget	• The practitioner greets each relative on arrival. • *The practitioner is mindful of potential breach to confidentiality*	• The person says they enjoyed their meal • The person is satisfied with sleep • The family feel involved in their relative's care

PROTOCOLS

Process criteria can be written as *Protocols* help to ensure consistency of 'best repose' to particular patients' needs. This is more so when 'best' practice has been researched and recommended by the National Institute of Clinical excellence [NICE]. Hence there must be good reason to deviate from their recommendations. Protocols are guides rather than prescriptions. Every situation is viewed on its particular circumstance requiring the practitioner to judge the appropriate response.

TRIGGERS FOR STANDARDS

The decision to construct a Standard of care can be triggered by any number of factors. This might be a complaint from a patient or a family member, a practitioner observing something, information suggesting other ways of doing things, or linked to implementing a new innovation or change in practice.

For example, the nutrition standard[4] emanated from observing that a person did not have a glass of water at hand at lunchtime. This led to constructing the standard 'Persons can enjoy a nutritious meal'. The trigger for a standard concerning sleep was appreciating that a person preferred to sleep in an armchair rather than in bed.

MONITORING TECHNIQUES

Monitoring criteria tools are designed to be integral within everyday practice – notably observational techniques such as scanning and spotting and through asking direct questions. Scanning is a planned monitoring of the standard of care using a designed scan sheet. Spotting is opportunistic observation of criteria during the course of the day. Using a Visual Analogue Scale (VAS) is helped for person's to monitor the extent of their satisfaction with such aspects as sleep (as illustrated in Box 4.2) or the extent the person feels practitioners have involved them in decisions about their care (see Box 7.4). Using a VAS begs the question – 'what factors influenced your score?'

As the standards group meets monthly, scanning of standards is usually undertaken monthly or more frequently if the aspect practice is 'spotted' as failing its criteria.

STANDARD KEEPERS

A standard of care is 'kept' by an allocated practitioner, preferably a practitioner who has a particular interest in that aspect of care. All practitioners accept this responsibility so all are involved including care assistants, and the involved work pressure is shared.

The standard keeper manages an associated 'resource file' comprising relevant information to inform the standard. This involves regular scrutiny of journals (available in the hospital library) to keep up to date. A clinical leadership role is to keep abreast of all the standards to ensure they are kept up to date through monitoring and journal articles.

WHO SHOULD MONITOR?

Scheduled scanning of standards is organised by the standard keeper who reports the outcome to the standards group for action or revision as necessary.

Nursing students and visitors to the hospital are invited to monitor standards, as part of their teaching programme. This enables them to critically learn about aspects of care and experience the idea of living quality and give feedback to practitioners.

Monitoring criteria that involve asking patients or their families are best slipped into normal conversation as integral to caring. Questions that invite the participant's judgement on quality of care processes require sensitivity. Visitors may be especially reluctant to give negative feedback when caring is in progress (Nehring and Geach 1973). As such, questions are better designed as open questions rather than closed questions.

THE STANDARDS GROUP

The standards group meets every month for two hours to review existing standards and develop new ones chaired by the standards of care facilitator. This role is rotated through the primary and associate nurses. The group has eight members, all nursing staff. The meetings are sacrosanct, planned in advance to facilitate maximum attendance. Meetings are scheduled for 3 p.m. set to overlap the late shift. Potentially it is a quieter time of the day. I say potentially because anything could happen to shatter the order. Approximately half the group will attend in their own time. We invite other professionals to join the group as relevant to the topic.

CONSTRUCTING THE STANDARD ON CONFIDENTIALITY

As I noted in Chapter 4, bedside handover was implemented to involve patients in their care. The practitioner would always cue the patient to self-disclose, for example 'How are you this morning?' as an opening gambit encouraging participation.

Of course, it was not always so straightforward. One morning I observed the night associate nurse and primary nurse communicating at the bedside of one lady in a three-bedded ward. They stood at the foot of the bed as the night nurse informed the primary nurse. The primary nurse was a little deaf and so the night nurse spoke loudly – loud enough for the observer to hear at the end of the ward and loud enough for the other two patients to hear what was being said. The woman in the bed was also deaf. She was sitting up trying to listen to what was being spoken, not being involved as the protocol stated. Clearly the protocol had failed and confidentiality broken.

After I shared my reflection on this event at the standards group, the group concurred it was a pertinent focus for a standard of care. A draft standard was written that stated – 'Persons do not have confidential information disclosed accidentally'.

The group then used a flipchart to brainstorm and explore actual and potential influencing factors drawing on the practitioners' own experiences participating in bedside handovers (Box 7.2). The resultant standard was constructed (Box 7.3) together with a scanning sheet to monitor the process and outcome criteria (Box 7.4).

The crux of appreciating confidentiality is to determine the meaning of 'public space' as set out in the UKCC code of professional conduct on confidentiality (UKCC 1987).[5] The group agreed that shared ward areas are public spaces and hence the practitioner should not voice things about the patient's care without the patient's permission that others might overhear. As

BOX 7.2 BRAINSTORMING RELEVANT FACTORS AROUND CONFIDENTIALITY

- Do patients want to be involved in bedside handover?
- In tune with our holistic vision?
- Shift of culture – old habits die hard, staff not committed to new pattern
- Pressure of time?
- Patients who are deaf but want to be involved?
- Where notes are stored and notes left open
- Professional responsibility – NMC code of ethics on confidentiality
- Is the bedside handover protocol adequate?
- How to monitor?
- Informing research and theory?
- Practitioner development (considering the trigger nature)

BOX 7.3 STANDARD STATEMENT: PERSONS DO NOT HAVE CONFIDENTIAL INFORMATION DISCLOSED ACCIDENTLY

Structure criteria

1. Persons' rights to confidentiality are set out in the hospital information booklet.
2. Orientation for new and existing staff to include teaching session on confidentiality and communication.
3. Notes stored in holders at foot of the person's bed.

Process criteria

1. The primary nurses discuss with each person/family the way nurses handover care and rights of confidentiality on admission.
2. All staff in such a way to ensure information about patients is not disclosed accidently by:
   - Nurses handover according to walk-round protocol (see Box 4.5)
   - To avoid careless stalk inside and outside the hospital
   - Mindful of inquiry and to whom information about the patient's care is disclosed
   - Leaving notes open

Outcome criteria (see scan sheet)

1. The person controls disclosure at bedside
2. The person feels involved in the handover
3. No accidental breach of confidentiality occurs at any time.

such, the bedside handover protocol stated that any patient unable or unwilling to engage in the bedside handover, were not talked about at the bedside.

Nursing students were asked to shadow the walk-round hand-over to monitor the standard and give practitioners feedback. As you might imagine, such scrutiny prompted practitioners to be more mindful of respecting confidentiality.

BOX 7.4 CONFIDENTIALITY SCAN SHEET

Standard statement: Persons do not have confidential information disclosed accidently

Date...............Observed by..................................1

No.	Observed action	Score/Scale 1........................10 1 = least agreement 10 = most agreement
1	Persons are involved in the hand-over of their care	
2	The person controls the disclosure of information concerning themselves	
3	Nurses do not talk about the patient outside the patient's listening	
4	No accidental breach of confidentiality occurs	
5	Person's notes are not left open in a public space	
	Ask each person (as able):	
6	'Do you think your nurses always treat what they know about your health-illness in a confidential manner?' (Sinha and Scherera 1987)	

THE VALUE OF STANDARDS OF CARE

Burford practitioners constructed 24 standards of care. Standards of care are dynamic, constantly being monitored and reviewed to ensure they reflect quality of care and that practice development is always at the forefront of Burford practice.

Constructing standards of care is worth every penny of staff time because of its significant benefits for any practice setting mindful of providing effective holistic practice especially those areas of practice that are often overlooked.

In summary Standards of care offer:

- A quality assurance process
- A way to integrate quality as part of everyday practice
- A framework for developing specific aspects of clinical practice
- A way for practitioners to demonstrate professional responsibility and

Accountability to develop and ensure effective holistic practice

- A change and resource management model
- A way of connecting values with practice
- A process of team learning
- A way to challenge 'normal' practice and solve unsatisfactory practice

CLINICAL AUDIT

Clinical audit enables practitioners across disciplines to collaborate and demonstrate professional responsibility to reflect on and gain insight through examination of specific situations. It has the same remit as guided reflection yet as a process of peer review. The intent is to improve practice (Clinical Audit in the NHS 1996). It is an opportunity for inter-disciplinary team learning to reflect and improve practice to answer two fundamental questions:

- Did the patient/family receive best care?
- Do we know what best care is?

Clinical audit is essentially a professional rather than an organisational activity. However, it may be difficult to distinguish between the two, given the organisation's concern with quality. As the Clinical Audit in the NHS (1996:4) notes –

> *Practitioners are only likely to become involved where they retain a clear sense of ownership of the process of audit and feel it is a safe environment for discussing sensitive details about their professional practice without the fear of provoking management sanction or civil litigation.*

IT WORKS LIKE THIS

A practitioner prepares and presents an overview of the patient's care. At Burford, I adapted the Model for Structured Reflection into a clinical audit tool (Box 7.5) The primary focus of review is on the specific event as an objective whereby the practitioners involved can stand back and consider whether best practice was realised and if not, why not, and how might it be done better if a similar situation arose, taking into account all influencing factors.

BOX 7.5 MODEL FOR REFLECTIVE INQUIRY

Influencing factors	The specific clinical event	Outcomes
• Did practitioners act for the best? (ethics) • Did practitioners act in tune with best practice? (empirics) • What factors influenced the situation? (environmental and personal)	How did practitioners: • grasp and interpret the situation? • plan response ? • actually respond? • judge the efficacy of response ?	Given a similar situation: • How might practitioners respond more effectively? • What factors might constrain practitioners and how might these be overcome? | | V What insights do we draw?

(Adapted from Johns 2022)

The review is led by the person's primary nurse, who summarises what insights have been gained to inform future practice. The situation is subsequently reviewed for impact (or not) at the next Clinical Audit review (every two months).

In summary, clinical audit is a formal, reflective, inter-disciplinary team learning session that reflects objectively on the situation rather than on the practitioners involved. A useful reflective ploy is to ask those practitioners not involved in the situation – 'what would you have done in this particular situation?', and to ask practitioners who were involved – 'what would you have done differently given the situation again?' both questions intending to open a creative space where these perspectives can be explored towards consensus.

SUMMARY

Living quality is the breathing heart of holistic practice because it requires the practitioner to be mindful of being and realising holistic practice moment by moment. Becoming mindful is achieved through communicative competence and the therapeutic team supplemented by guided reflection, standards of care and clinical audit. Living quality is creative and dynamic, meaning that no aspect of practice becomes routine or taken for granted.

The next three chapters are accounts written by Burford practitioners reflecting on 'living' holistic practice through the Burford NDU holistic model.

NOTES

1 This definition has remained unchanged (DOH September 2022).

2 QUALPACS see M. A. Wandelt and J. W. Ager, *Quality Patient Care Scale* (New York: Appleton-Century-Crofts, 1974)

Phaneuf nursing audit see Phaneuf, M. (1976). *The Nursing Audit: Self-regulation in nursing practice* (2nd ed). New York: Appleton-Century-Crofts.

3 Standards of care were initially developed as an approach to quality and clinical practice development by the Royal College of Nursing Standards of Care project.

4 The nutrition standard of care outcome criteria scanning sheet can be viewed in Table 21.1 (page 238) in Johns C (2022) A system to enable practitioners to live and ensure quality. In *Becoming a reflective practitioner (sixth edition)* Wiley Blackwell, Oxford.

5 See Nursing and Midwifery Council (NMC) Code of professional conduct 2015.

REFERENCES

Department of Health (1996) *Clinical audit in the NHS*. HMSO, London.

Department of Health (2022) *Clinical governance*. HMSO, London.

Johns C (2022) A system to enable practitioners to live and ensure quality. In *Becoming a reflective practitioner* (sixth edition) (Ed. C Johns) Wiley Blackwell, Oxford p233–234. (Figure 21.1).

Nehring V and Geach B (1973) Why they don't complain: patient's evaluation of their care. *Nursing Outlook* 21(5); 317–21.

Sinha L and Scherera K (1987) Quality assurance: ask the patient. *Nursing Times* 83(45); 40–42.

PART 2

Practitioner Accounts

Caring as Mutual Empowerment: Working with the BNDU Model at Burford

CHAPTER 8

Lyn Sutherland

I shall illustrate and critique my engagement with the Burford NDU model through using a case study of work with a patient and her family whom I was privileged to be her primary nurse.

JOAN

Joan came to Burford hospital after surgery 'for a few days convalescence' according to the transfer letter which her family handed to us on her arrival. She died five weeks later. She had been ill for just the three months of her 66 years.

During those last weeks, Joan and her family moved from a position of fear, disbelief, conspiracy and hopelessness to the point where, in spite of their sadness, they were able to share fully in the experience of death as a healing in itself rather than as a failure.

HER ADMISSION TO BURFORD

Joan was exhausted on arrival, having travelled by car with her husband and daughter-in-law only seven days after her operation. Unable to keep her eyes open, she climbed into bed with hardly a word and slept at once. Only her tiredness, and slight unsteadiness of gait, and the new incision on her partly shaved head, indicated that she was unwell. As the primary nurse assigned to facilitate Joan's care I sat and had a drink with Tom and Val while they began to tell me their story. Val did much of the talking with Tom's acquiescence and occasional additions. The salient points gradually emerged.

> *They told us she's got a grade 4 tumour – that's very malignant. We know they haven't cleared it all away and that it may grow again. So they might have to give her radiotherapy. She may not live for very long, possibly only a few months. We think she knew it was a tumour before she was admitted to have it removed,, because she had a brother who died of a brain tumour years ago. As soon as they confirmed it she started to go downhill. So although we give her truthful answers to anything she asks us we're not directly telling her anything. She's not asked much at all.*

Holistic Practice in Healthcare: The Burford NDU Person-centred Model, Second Edition. Edited by Christopher Johns.

After I asked for a few biographical details Tom and Val left taking the hospital's information brochure with them. Having been made aware of the open visiting policy they promised Joan they would return later.

By this point I had spent about 40 minutes listening to Val and Tom and about 2 minutes with Joan. To what avail? I had virtually nothing on paper, no neat assessment tool filled with an odd word or two under the headings. 'No one will read it if it's too lengthy', I thought. Yet I felt comfortable about this. Why? I had not communicated to any great extent with Joan and I had little information about her condition and its impact on her activities of living.

My experience prior to arriving at Burford had been exclusively in the acute field where I would have required such factual information as soon after Joan's admission as possible. A mindset of 'I must get this out of the way' as a task to complete.

I can only answer this by referring to the Burford model. By the time I was appointed as a primary nurse, the model had been established to guide practice. The vision had been sent to me as part of the information I received on applying to Burford. I felt instinctively comfortable with it in spite of not 'owning' it by contributing to its evolution. On first encountering the assessment tool I found it difficult to know what to do with it. My initial attempts involved 'filling in' the answers to the cue questions as they appeared on the printed sheet. I felt awkward and threatened that it appeared to be expected that I would expose myself and make myself vulnerable by writing about my own feelings.[1] It did not act as an aide-memoire for all the things I needed to know about a patient's physical condition, and didn't I felt help me structure information useful to other hospital colleagues.[2]

By the time Joan was admitted I had been at Burford 5 months. I felt much more familiar with the model. It had become a part of me how I approached my practice. I no longer had to refer directly to the documents in order to recall their premises. The way of thinking and assessing suggested by the model was beginning to feel more natural.[3]

So it was easier for me to accept that Joan's need for sleep was far more important than my need to gather information. That could wait till later. The vision not only guides me to view Joan holistically as 'greater than the sum of her parts', but to see her from her social situation. Val and Tom willingly gave me much valuable information and the above notes form only an outline of the rich store of knowledge not only about Joan but about themselves, and the frightening uncharted scenario they all faced.

At the end of our time together, a picture was emerging against the background of the model that indicated a great deal about what was happening to this family. The doctor's letter was not needed to tell me about her right occipital lobe glioma because Val described how the tumour showed itself – the abnormal sight, balance difficulties and headaches that it had caused Joan. And how quickly that had all happened. So the health event that had necessitated medical care was plain without need for a precise technical definition at this stage.

HER FAMILY

It became evident that Joan and her husband Tom had a close family, and a largely ordered contended life, with the key members living within a few miles of one another. Their son and wife Val, had two children of primary school age. Their daughter Ann worked in a local shop. They had many friends in the area. Val and Ann's unwavering support for Joan and for each other was noticeable from the beginning, and it was evident that they were prepared to turn their lives over completely to caring for Joan for as long as necessary.

However, this paints too simplistic a picture. They were also upset, shocked, frightened of the future, angry, disbelieving, and desperately protective of Joan. They wanted to explain to me in detail what she could do or could not do for herself, and in particular they wanted to control what she was told about her illness and prognosis. Much of their own fear was evidenced in the way they emphasised that she would not be able to cope with the knowledge, that telling her anything about it would no doubt ensure a faster deterioration, and they desperately wanted the staff to collude in all this. I felt admiration and respect for the way they were all pulling together and supporting each other. I felt I could help them in the difficulties they faced with my knowledge of palliative care, and the many experiences I had shared with other families as one of the members approached death. I knew that at the time the first thing I needed to do was to enable them to express their fears, which without defusing would lead to a damaging conspiracy of silence which could overshadow and taint all else.

JOAN'S CARE BY FAMILY AND NURSING STAFF

Later in the evening Joan woke and the full character of her Northern accent, unusual in the Cotswolds became obvious. Naturally gregarious as a rule, she did not really feel up to chatting to other patients, even though she was quite lucid and happy to talk about her background and family to me. Not having a great appetite, a cup of tea sufficed for supper, and afterwards I removed her sutures, due out that day.

Her unsteadiness was very evident when she launched herself towards the bathroom. She needed to urinate frequently due to taking dexamethasone. This alone did not control her headaches, for which she was prescribed codeine phosphate. Her bowels had been opened that morning. Once she had settled again, it became clear that she could manage herself in the bed and help with pressure relief did not seem to be needed at least at this time. She seemed contented to be in the less busy atmosphere that a community hospital can provide, and relieved to be nearer home.

Over the next few days, we found that most of what was needed to make Joan's stay with us as comfortable as possible was willingly provided by her family. She continued to need a great deal of sleep, and her own bedding from home soon made an appearance as she found this much more acceptable than standard hospital provision. All the family and a number of friends spent time with her at intervals during the day, and either Val or Ann would help her with a bath at some point daily. They brought food she fancied from home, and she began to feel up to dressing.

This of course meant that a great deal of advice, explanation and support for the family carers was needed from the nursing staff. Problems that needed tacking during this period included careful attention to the nature of her different pains with appropriate pharmacological manipulation and concurrent intervention to alleviate constipation. Allowance also had to be made for her unpredictable mobility due to the effects of increased intra-cranial pressure on her balance and sight. Joan's mucous membranes became very dry. As she slept so much her fluid intake was not high and she didn't feel like eating much.

The Burford vision stresses that care is centred around the needs of the person and that person continues to be a person within their community. For Joan and her family, the hospital became a natural extension of their own homes, and they cared for her almost exclusively whilst not shunning help from staff when they did need it. The model enabled me to plan care that laid emphasis of care for the family both as givers with support to care for Joan and as receivers to be cared for. Far from being passive in her dependency, Joan evidently gave her family much in return.

I felt comfortable about enabling the family's control of what was happening without feeling that I had abdicated my responsibility with the attendant guilt of not 'doing' enough for them. I was involved and working 'with' them. With my associate nurse colleagues we were continually re-evaluating the situation in the light of the cue questions responding with concern and poise within the shifting tides of their unfolding experience.

Throughout the initial days of Joan's stay, the family remained hesitant about talking to Joan about her diagnosis. Two things precipitated movement towards more open communication, Firstly, Joan began to ask more about what was happening. She began to explore the nature of her illness with me so that when eventually she asked a direct question during a talk with one of the GPs, he was able to confirm that the operation had been to remove a part of the cancer. He stressed that knowing what was wrong would help her fight it. This felt important because at this time Joan was talking very much in terms of the future when she would have recovered.

It was hard for the family to know that Joan and asked and been told this. As a consequence, much work was needed throughout this time to help them through their resurfaced anger, disbelief and constant search to know how best to respond to Joan. Secondly, the date set for Joan's out-patient appointment in the radiotherapy department was imminent. I felt it was imperative that the family should understand that Joan's diagnosis and prognosis were likely to be discussed in full at this time so that all would be in a position to enable her to make the best decision about her treatment.

Plans were made for Joan to go home and spend the weekend before the appointment with a degree of anxiety and apprehension as well as eager anticipation. Saturday went well but on Sunday morning Ann phoned with a story of deterioration; vomiting, increased drowsiness, inability to swallow fluids or take her medication. They returned to hospital later that day.

Medication review was not entirely successful. The following morning revealed an obvious left-sided weakness. A joint decision was made that she should still attend the out-patient appointment tomorrow. With close liaison between ourselves, the department and the ambulance service, Joan and her family were able to keep this long awaited appointment whilst ensuring an acceptable degree of comfort for Joan despite the distance involved.

There was an atmosphere of profound relief when she returned. Joan had been told that there was no need for her to receive radiotherapy and that nothing more could be done for the present except to increase her dexamethasone. Her relatives had been told that her prognosis was only a few weeks and that radiotherapy would not change the course of her illness and that increasing the dexamethasone might help to give her a short period of 'normal' life to enjoy together.

A further development came after this evening when another GP visited. Joan asked him directly if she was going to die. He confirmed this saying that her family knew too.

HER REALISATION OF DYING

This heralded a new phase in Joan's care. It was necessary to realign our approach to explore her feelings now her previously unspoken fears of dying had been confirmed. Although effective pain relief and symptom control were still of utmost importance, the 'work' with Joan and her family was much more. The cue questions with their emphasis on 'helping', 'feeling' and 'supporting' ensured I was in tune with the emerging situation.

Tom and each member of the family needed help to gauge how to respond to Joan now that the truth was known and acknowledged by all. There was still a great desire on all sides that Joan's care to be based at home as possible yet with great apprehension. Daytime visits home both planned and spontaneous proved to be the best solution with everyone aware that the decision to return home lay with them, not with us. This gave Joan the confidence to remain overnight on two occasions enabling her and Tom to have time completely alone.

Joan openly explored her thoughts and feelings with me that I recorded in her narrative notes. Writing enabled me to reflect more deeply on our conversations, enabling me to work through my own feelings and helping me to remain poised and keep things in perspective. She told me she would like to go to church and the vicar visited several times. Joan's level of orientation, consciousness and ability fluctuated remarkably widely at this time and this dictated the tenor of our conversations and her daily activity and responsiveness to staff and visitors.

After this period of readjustment and regrouping Joan began to deteriorate rapidly. The balance of care shifted as the family members increasingly sought for help with her direct physical care. Joan's pain management was changed to continuous subcutaneous diamorphine. She had become completely dependent on family and staff gradually deteriorating until Joan was deeply unconscious, hyperpyrexic and tachycardic with her limbs held in stiff extension. Her urine output was still significant and catheterisation became necessary to maintain dignity and comfort.

One afternoon as I was attending Joan with Val, she suddenly woke up and asked for a drink and sit up. Although unable to articulate clearly, it was obvious she understood all that was being spoken and responding as best as she could. Some of the family were able to enjoy this time with her, until just a few hours later she became unrousable again. She died the following afternoon amongst her family and belongings in her room which, although part of the hospital, had truly become part of their home.

REFLECTION ON JOAN'S CARE

Initially I experienced a sense of disappointment and regret when Joan died. I asked myself why I felt like that? I believe it was because I had not been able to share in her final hours as I was off-duty at the time and that privilege lay with one of my colleagues. Nor was I free to attend her funeral although I spoke with the family that morning. Given that we could not change the relentless progress of her illness we had nevertheless we had been able to care in such a way that her family were able to continue their grieving from a strong position where their own healing could begin.

Reviewing Joan's notes revealed her journey from admission to her death in just a few weeks, from feelings of devastation and despair through questioning, anxiety and anger to a place of contentment and acceptance alongside their sadness. There is much comment on the dialogue between myself and colleagues that charts this progression, where practical matters and symptom management blend into the whole human story.

REFLECTION ON THE BURFORD NDU MODEL

The assessment tool comprising a set of cues to tune me into the hospital's vision certainly focused me on what I consider the effective caring for Joan and her family. Prior to coming to Burford, my knowledge of nursing models had been very limited and I doubt that

I understood their significance in guiding a practitioner to relate to and care for a patient. Coming into contact with the different way of thinking made explicit by the model enabled me to start breaking away from the lip service to individualised and routinised approach to patients which is so common and which I had been socialised over so many years. So why do I think this?

UNDERSTANDING THE PHILOSOPHY

Firstly, the language and format are accessible. There are no words in either the vision or assessment tool that require a specialist understanding or explanation. There are no complicated diagrams to interpret. Johns (1991) gives an example of how one of the cue questions had to be changed at an early stage because a problem arose with wording (and therefore a concept) which was not immediately meaningful. He comments too that 'the complex construction of many models makes them intimidating and difficult to use' whereas Damant (1988) notes Baer's argument that a profession needs its own language if it is to successfully articulate and pass on knowledge and skills. In my opinion, the Burford model does this exquisitely. Wright (1990) questions whether new language is genuinely needed to express new ideas or whether it is employed to lend credence to academics and theorists. As a nurse whose own education is only slowly increasing, I appreciate it when academics can make their ideas available to practitioners. However, in spite of the availability of the Burford model, I was initially at a loss to know quite what to 'do' with the assessment tool. But as I settled in with guidance from my colleagues I was encouraged to find myself beginning to understand how the model was leading me to care for patients (and here read persons) from a different perspective, despite my lack of theoretical knowledge background and practical experience of living out the concepts the model embraces.

Because the emphasis is centred on feelings and the total picture of the person's situation rather than just on their presenting physical needs, it forced me to move away from a need to find things out, fill things in, and get things done as soon as possible in an orderly fashion. It forced me[4] to start to listen to the persons' stories, what they were saying was important to them and then to plan care with them from this basis. Duke and Copp (1992) note 'the caring aspect of nursing becomes hidden, often among tasks or defined in the context of tasks'.

It gradually became a welcome release for me, rather than an abandonment into a void, to be able to think through my approach to a person's care within this new framework. Task identification related to physical need was no longer the raison d'etre of assessment. Although at first I found myself going back to Roper et al.'s (1980) headings to make myself feel secure that I had not missed something that was physically important, I did not need to do this for long. Dialogue with colleagues and reading about the emergence of the vision and the roots of the cue questions helped me enormously in enabling a deeper sensitivity towards the model and confidence in its use.

I said that one of the things that drew me to work at Burford was an 'instinctive' feel that I could practise within the vision. Now, more than that, I feel it articulates ideas that I had in my own mind about the way I wanted to work with people but were very difficult to realise in my previous posts.[5] So the spelling out of these ideas gave me permission to try and realise them more successfully than previously. Of course the reflective learning culture of Burford facilitated this conversion.

VALUING THE NURSE

The worth and contribution of nurses as persons is not merely recognised but emphasised as an essential part of the person's care. Even now, nurses are still more used to acting in a service role and the completion of tasks rather than working in more responsible ways with and alongside persons. The model not only refers to the patient as a person but also implicitly the nurse as a person. Because the words 'patient' and 'nurse' are not used, it draws away from condemning either to traditional roles. Instead one is led to think and question from a human point of view of one person learning to help another – the one with special needs at the time and the other with special knowing to assist. As the vision emphasises care is a mutual process – hence I became open to learning from the person.

Prompting one to think – 'How can I help this person?' 'How is this person feeling?' and 'How does this person make me feel?' – these cues cannot fail to provoke a response which leads to using not only one's specialised knowing but also one's personal qualities giving credence to Pearson's (1991) comment that 'the nurse has the right to be honoured as a unique individual as well'. Being acknowledged as a person gave me permission to see the other as a person. This equation had a profound impact on the quality of my relationships that emerged and the quality of care that ensued.

REFLECTION ON 'CARING'

The word 'care' features repeatedly within the holistic vision:

- 'we believe that care is centred around'
- 'trust is developed that enhances care'
- 'effective patient care and comfort is the first priority of the hospital'
- 'an integral part of community care'
- 'a therapeutic environment that can only enhance patient care'

'Care' has also featured frequently in my reflection in this case study. The model tunes you into thinking about the nature of caring and thus into one of the biggest debates in nursing today. It is similar to words such as 'professional' and 'reassurance' which are constantly used but hardly ever defined by practising nurses. Pearson (1991) considers the association of care with compassion noting that both care and compassion are words rooted in Celtic meaning 'to cry out with' and 'to enter into'. He also quotes Benner, who in 1985 wrote of her view that 'caring provides empowerment rather than control'. Malin and Teasdale (1991) suggest the opposite; that there is a tension between caring and empowerment. They discuss Griffin's opinion that the very act of caring removes autonomy from a patient. Morse (1991) feels that commitment may be a more appropriate term to use than caring. She is speaking here of the nurse-patient relationship suggesting that it is impossible to consider the nature of caring without addressing the complexities of this concept to.

These are just a few of the many writers who have considered the subject of caring whereby a difference in views is evident. If caring is one of the chief purposes of our work as nurses, then it is imperative that we attend to this debate, reflect on it ourselves and begin to make sense of it in our own practices. The Burford model makes it impossible not to do so, for in responding to a person in the light of the cue questions set against the background of the Burford vision the debate becomes part of everyday practice rather than locked up in theoretical discourse.[6]

In Joan's case, caring for her meant a continuous sensitive response to the enormous changes happening to her and her family, an opening and exploration of myself and my knowing to respond to their needs, to become available to them, progressing with them and certainly empowering them.

I wonder how they would describe their experience of being cared for, both then and now with hindsight; whether they would identify with the way I described what happened, whether they would unconsciously use a similar vocabulary, or words that mean similar things in 'lay' terms. I doubt whether they realised that the way I tried to help them was framed within a model and I don't think they would give it a second thought. But although I have not formally evaluated their perceptions of the care they received, all informal feedback (chance meetings of staff with family members in the village) indicate that they hold a very positive view of it.

BECOMING A REFLECTIVE PRACTITIONER

One of the important things about working at Burford is becoming a reflective practitioner. This involved keeping a diary as a means of reflecting on my experiences with persons and colleagues. Anything that emerges as significant to practice can be reflected on and recorded. During monthly supervision (guided reflection) sessions with my clinical leader and guide I felt safe to explore these experiences recorded in my diary. In the relating of these experiences and by engaging in a relevant theory, I learnt from both the examination of dissatisfying experiences and celebration of successful strategies. These reflective skills needed to be learnt and practised and were not initially easy to acquire, but it gradually became second nature to reflect throughout the day, not just on writing a diary.

I firmly believe that starting to learn to be a reflective practitioner myself has been one of the most important parts of my nursing life. The skills of perception and analysis, the sensitivity, intuition and willingness to be genuine required to be a reflective practitioner are complementary to, indeed, essentially the same as those needed to utilise the model as a basis for clinical practice.

REFLECTION ON CLINICAL LEADERSHIP

The role of the clinical leader in the role of guide plays a powerful part in honing the skills of a primary nurse. In this case, the clinical leader was also the driving force behind the evolving of the model. It was difficult for me to ascertain to what extent other staff had been involved, and the degree to which the model was truly the Burford model or whether it should more aptly be named the Johns' model. Why should it not be? There are many precedents to this – virtually every other model I know of is named after the person rather than a place and seems to be rooted firmly in that person's work over some years. It is not given to everyone to be able to study at a higher level, and in developing any field of study there will be those whose gift it is to explore concepts and push boundaries. Whilst not minimising the motivating effect of working with such a person, and the influence that having such a strong leader can have, it is important to note that the nature of practice at Burford obliges each practitioner to constantly reflect on the work going on from their own knowledge and experience. So I did feel able to question those aspects of working with the model that I did not initially understand, learning through everyday events and dialogue with colleagues, through personal reflection and through supervision.

Working in a small unit also means that each person's contribution to the life and welfare of the hospital and all the people involved is unique, intensely personal and comes under close scrutiny. It is inevitable that each person's practice will in itself influence and mould the tools being used to frame care.

So, in one sense it is the Johns' model, in that much of the background work is his. In another sense, however, it is impossible for the model to develop without committing it to practice, and so it becomes owned and moulded too by those who use it.

POST BURFORD

Since leaving Burford it has been necessary to use other models. However, my practice has continued to be influenced by my experience using the Burford model. I became aware of this vividly one day during my district nurse training. I was asked to assess Mabel, an elderly lady who had multiple medical problems complicated by difficult social circumstances. On the day I made my first visit, I was feeling low and unconfident in myself, and my own concerns were still uppermost in my mind as I knocked on her door. Meeting this very agitated and unwell lady for the first time in her own home, crowded with paraphernalia associated with and extended family across the generations living in too small a space, threw me completely. My first instinct was to find an excuse to leave and try to get some help for me! My second was to reach for a tight assessment structure with which I could marshal some sense of order out of the muddled situation, and gain some sort of control. I wanted to be told specific problems for which I would feel safe to prescribe definite actions. However, my socialisation as a nurse prevented me from giving into the first option, and I felt instinctively that the second option would crush Mabel rather than succeed in finding out what was really bothering her. So I tried to concentrate on her story. As I did, so I felt my feelings of helplessness diminish as I paid attention to what she was trying to articulate. I slowly began to think more rationally – 'who is this person?' 'what do I need to know to be able to help her?' As I continued to listen, actively now and with renewing confidence, the familiar Burford cue questions formed the background to the way I began to respond to her. I was using the Burford model. I know that the Burford model will be helping me to nurse for many years to come.[7]

NOTES

1 This is a powerful confession of how practitioners defend themselves from the emotional side of practice. The cue – 'how do I feel about the person' does not require a concrete answer – it is just a cue to open the practitioner to their feelings, not necessarily to write about them. It shows how conditioned practitioners can become to filling in boxes 'because it is expected to fill them in'.

2 I suspect that Lyn's comment is a fairly typical reflection that practitioners might make faced with the Burford model after using other seemingly more structured models. It reflects how the mind becomes accustomed to viewing the world in a restricted way. Why do practitioners need a very structured approach? What are they fearful of? Is it making a mistake or missing something as Sutherland suggests?

3 Lyn reflects how the model has become natural for her after 5 months, a more instinctive response to it that has liberated her, reinforcing my assertion how over time through experience the cues become internalised and a natural way for seeing and responding to practice.

4 Note Lyn's use of the word 'forced' – reflecting how using the cues cut across her previous experience of assessment.

5 I am certain that this comment resonates with many practitioners- that somewhere in their mind they want to practice holistic nursing but have not been able to either articulate that or work in practice settings that subscribe to holistic practice, brewing dissatisfaction and frustration that ultimately leads to burn-out. What you might describe as 'unhealthy nursing'.

6 Lyn alludes to the notion that caring is known as something lived and reflected on in practice rather than a theoretical debate and that if practitioners want to care they must first grasp an idea of what holistic practice looks like, find structures to facilitate it in practice, gain the necessary support to reflect on it, and in doing so increasingly come to live caring as a lived reality. This is the essence of the Burford model. It was created to facilitate living holistic practice.

7 Lyn notes how the Burford model remained an influence in her later work as a district nurse. However, when I asked her why she did not use the Burford model in her district nursing, she replied that she was expected to use another model irrespective of its value in seeing and working with patients. Her comment leads me to draw two conclusions: firstly, how practice settings impose models of practitioners, and secondly, how passive practitioners are in accepting such imposition especially when other models may be more suitable. It reflects the organisational dominance of practice over a professional approach. Lyn commented further that part of the problem was that her district nursing practice had not been defined and hence neither practice nor the use of nursing model had direction or meaning.

REFERENCES

Damant M (1988) Innovations in assessment. *Journal of District Nursing* 6(9); 9–12.

Duke S and Copp G (1992) Hidden nursing. *Nursing Times* 88(17); 40–2.

Johns C (1991) The Burford nursing development unit holistic model of nursing practice. *Journal of Advanced Nursing* 16; 1090–8.

Malin N and Teasdale K (1991) Caring versus empowerment: considerations for nursing practice. *Journal of Advanced Nursing* 16; 657–62.

Morse J (1991) Negotiating commitment and involvement in the nurse-patient relationship. *Journal of Advanced Nursing* 16; 455–68.

Pearson A (1991) Taking up the challenge: the future for therapeutic nursing. In *Nursing as Therapy* (Eds. R McMahon and A Pearson) Chapman and Hall, London.

Roper N, Logan W, and Tierney A (1980) *Elements of nursing* Churchill Livingstone, Edinburgh.

Wright S (1990) Useless theory or aids to practice? In *Models of Nursing 2* (Eds. B Kershaw and J Salvage) Scutari Press, Harrow.

Discovering the Art of Nursing: Using the BNDU Model at Burford

CHAPTER 9

Roger Cowell

During an early supervision session[1] with Chris Johns, I was very excited to share a quote from Oliver Sacks's book *Awakenings* because it spoke so much to me about using the Burford model.

> *We must come down from our position as 'objective observers and meet our patients face-to-face: we must meet them in a sympathetic and imaginative encounter, for it is only in the context of such collaboration, a participation, relation, that we can hope to learn anything about how they are. (Sacks 1990:7–8)*[2]

Sacks's words accord closely with the way I wanted to nurse, the relationships I wanted to achieve with my patients and colleagues, and with the vision and model practised at Burford.

Frankly, in my early days at Burford, I struggled to grasp and make sense of the model in my relationships. I had read books with related approaches such as Awakenings [noted above] and Carl Rogers writing about the therapeutic relationship. Now, more than a year later, I remain engaged in that struggle but from a different perspective. This new perspective is captured by the following quotation by Maynard Keynes in his 'Preface to general theory' –

> *The very difficulty lies not in the new ideas but in escaping from the old ones, which ramify, for those brought up as most of have been, into every corner of our minds. (Cited by Sacks 1990: xiv)*

In my early days, I wrote in my diary

> *Where am I with my colleagues? We don't know each other well enough to be much more than a 'harmonious team', that is, we are not yet giving each other much feedback – that I want to give and get.*

I also reflected on my assessment of patient care and tentative use of the cue questions within the holistic model.

> *These are hard to grasp in that in a large acute ward the principal questions are for priorities of physical care where social and psychological need are almost identified by chance. Its hard not to ask patients directly rather than bear the questions in mind as cues...in my previous practice I reflected on my practice more than many of my colleagues but in comparison with now was not very much!*[3]

Holistic Practice in Healthcare: The Burford NDU Person-centred Model, Second Edition. Edited by Christopher Johns.

ESCAPE

The turning point in my escape story from old ideas, was a very painful afternoon of 'group reflection' with my colleagues.[4] They told me that they perceived me as unsupportive and unforthcoming of feedback. That night I noted in my reflective diary

What do I feel tonight?

Distress	threat
Sorrow	dismay
Loss	sadness
Pain more	threat
Isolation	insecurity
Dislocation	puzzlement

I recognised then that my low mood about myself was getting in the way of giving and receiving feedback with both my patients and colleagues. This cathartic experience made it possible to ask myself more or less the same questions of myself as the model's cue questions to enable me to confront myself – 'who am I'? that proved essential to enable me to nurse my patients effectively in tune with the Burford vision.[5]

In my diary I had reflected on a number of particular patients. My commitment to a holistic vision and ensuing model for practice brings me naturally to reflect on my patients and their humanity.

MADGE BROWN: FACILITATING SHIFTS IN ATTITUDE TO PROMOTE CARE OF A 'DIFFICULT' PATIENT

My first response to Madge was sheer panic. She arrived at the hospital on a Friday afternoon. She was far more dependent than I had anticipated from conversations from nurses from her referring hospital. She was 73, nearly blind, an insulin-dependent diabetic, heavy, with both legs amputated just below the knee, had recently suffered a stroke that left her with a dense left hemiplegia, and had recently been diagnosed with carcinoma of the rectum.

I felt she would require more nursing attention than we could give, so, after making this judgement, I informed the GP what my colleagues and I felt. The GP responded very personally – 'are you saying you can't cope, that you haven't enough staff?' I replied – 'we don't have enough resources to care for her and could not see what the outcome would be.' The GP replied 'Well, that's your problem not mine.[6]'

A number of other staff expressed their opinion that it was ridiculous for us to look after her and inappropriate for her to be in a community hospital.[7] That was also my opinion at first, but the GP's stinging response for my request for support spurred me to look at this person as a human being not just an unwelcome burden on the workload.

Obviously physical resources such as the use of a 'Pegasus' mattress, a hoist and sling, made the management of Madge's care possible, even if still time-consuming. But it was establishing a relationship with Madge and her husband Bill, which led me and eventually my colleagues to define and achieve desirable outcomes of care prompted by the BNDU cues.

As the primary nurse I am caregiver and care planner. As such, my assessment is not merely a snapshot on admission but something continuous, reminiscent of Sacks's 'sympathetic and imaginative encounter'. So it was that whilst giving direct care, assisting her with breakfast one morning I broke through to Madge face-to-face. I wondered aloud if she would like to take the beaker of tea herself, take her cereal spoon and slices of toast from the plate. Her poor eyesight required my instruction where to feel for the food, whether she had filled her spoon, where her beaker was and where she could find the plate of toast. So it did not mean that I could attend to someone else. But it did mean that Madge discovered that she could still do things which neither the staff at the previous hospital nor her family had let her do. It was the BNDU model that prompted my questioning 'How did Madge feel?' I asked her what it was like to use the utensils now. She smiled and said 'it makes me feel human again'.

It is during the giving of such personal care that the BNDU model brings the cue questions repeatedly to mind. This was evident in another experience of working with Madge when a care assistant and I were helping Madge to change her position in bed, I asked her to move her legs to one side. She replied immediately 'You mean my stumps'. I challenged her with the suggestion that her legs were still her legs regardless of being partially amputated.

Such individual interactions do not necessarily affect the interactions of colleagues even if recorded. It was necessary to communicate the desired outcomes to Madge's family in a form that might facilitate their reflection on their relationship with Madge.

I prepared a Special Intervention (SI) sheet[8] describing the two incidents outlined above asking my colleagues to consistently follow my approach with utensils and to challenge Madge when she made comments suggesting low self-esteem. I asked my colleagues for feedback on how they felt when Madge made negative comments and how they responded to her. These were both recorded and given verbally.

After a few weeks, Madge was referring spontaneously and consistently to her legs and talking more to the nursing staff. Staff, including those who had been critical and sceptical of my decision to accept her for our care, made comments to me of their enjoyment of caring for Madge and their pleasure when Madge managed particularly well with some aspects of self-care.

CONTINUING ASSESSMENT WITH THE BNDU MODEL

I was mindful of Madge's health experience evolving through her stay working towards a scenario whereby Madge could be discharged. Bill was determined to care for her at home and despite limited availability of community care staff to support them, despite the obstruction and scepticism of some community personnel, and despite the added complication of 'cross-border' referral, a workable package was negotiated including flexible respite care. Madge was discharged and her and Bill's desire to be together was achieved. A post-discharge home visit conformed that the package was working well. Seeing Madge in her bedroom, in a hospital bed, with radio, television, and bedside telephone, near a window where she could hear birds outside, confirmed to me that her discharge was a success. Bill was coping well though Penny, the district nurse, who spent an hour of more daily with Madge found this a severe strain on her workload.

Respite care for one week varied between 4 and 8 weeks. As her carcinoma spread she experienced great pain, insomnia, increased anxiety and confusion. Despite medication she became agitated and suspicious of others. She was also intermittently unaware of whether she was at home or in hospital. At this time I asked Madge how she viewed the future. She said 'I don't think about it. It's too painful.'

It was upsetting for Bill and myself and colleagues to see her deteriorate. She was not the same Madge Brown we used to know. The BNDU model makes practitioners continually focus on themselves as individuals, and in this situation made me focus my concern and my colleagues' concerns on our feelings – through the BNDU cues:

'How must this person be feeling?'

'How does this person make me feel?'

In response to these cues, I discussed my perceptions of change with the associate nurses, care assistants, the district nurse and with Bill, so that we could share how we felt about Madge and reach some mutual appreciation of how best to care for her and support each other. The outpouring of feelings felt like grieving.

The cues open the tap on feelings that prior to working at Burford had not been an issue simply because I had kept an emotional distance from patients. This was no longer the case. Now who I am as a person was primary in the care I gave.

My concern for Madge and Bill was full blown and as a consequence I became absorbed in their suffering. The support of my colleagues she shared similar feelings was vital as was guidance in supervision to enable me to put my feelings into perspective and remain poised.

My care planning became collegial stemming from the belief within our hospital vision that recognises we are committed to involvement with our patients and with each other. Rather than running away from uncomfortable feelings, I could pay attention to them and deal with them appropriately as a significant determinant in our care. At times my colleagues confronted me with our difficulties in caring for Madge highlighting the need to continually dialogue and support each other.

Supporting Bill became increasingly significant in the light of these changes to Madge's condition. I constantly 'cued' him to share his feelings and thoughts concerning Madge's care to the point I suggested that if he decided he could no longer adequately care for Madge at home then she could come to Burford for terminal care. He was not sleeping much and was very tired and stressed but was determined to care for Madge at home until she died and in that he succeeded.

JOHNY ARTHUR

As with Madge and Bill, the BNDU model prompted (and reminded) me to view people as rounded individuals rather than as 'types', which I believe how I, in common with many nurses, viewed many patients in previous nursing environments, necessary to develop therapeutic relationships. This is illustrated with clarity in the development of my skills in portraying people on paper, as in my discharge letter for Johny Arthur to his new nursing home.

> *Mr Arthur was admitted to us for overnight observation. It was clear he had suffered a cerebral vascular accident, or at best a transient ischaemic attack. Over the following few days, Johny was very agitated and restless, and then deteriorated markedly but then a further recovery in cosnciousness. He exhibited a severe visual impairment – a right hemianopia – which is in no sense resolved, and which remains a puzzle and source of anxiety for him.*

According to his former landlady, Johny has been restless, anxious and agitated as long as she has known him, and these traits have been magnified by his stroke. At times, both I the early incident period and in the weeks and months since, he has been so agitated as to require major tranquillisers. He responds to calm, firm direction perhaps as a result of his military wartime experience, or, failing that, he may just be left to his own devices to calm down. He can be very variable in mood and response during each day and from day to day.

Johny has in many ways made a fine recovery physically. Sadly, however, Johny's anxiety has been accompanied by a tendency to talk quite extravagantly and inappropriately, and at great length. Sometimes he is painfully aware that he is talking nonsense, and it may be interspersed with genuine sense, and he may respond in a fully appropriate manner.

Johny had little insight into his illness for a long period of his stay with us, and this was at times a hindrance to his recovery and sometimes, in a sense, a kindness. But he has developed insights that are quite real and deep, for instance, see the photocopied Special Intervention sheet [see figure 4.1]. It has not always been easy to support and care for Johny. At times, he has been pleasant and at times frustrating, difficult and sad. Here is a man whose elife has been changed dramatically by this change to his health. I hope you will be able to accept him and value him as a person, a man of considerable depth, wit, and charm, with many other facets – in short, a human being like all of us.

When I shared this letter with colleagues they fedback that I had captured the essence of Johny's essence and care. I contrasted this with what I associate as a standard discharge letter that says something like 'thank you taking this pleasant gentleman'.

I prepared this portrait from the perceptive and detailed reflections in his notes. The use of narrative form and use of Special Intervention sheets for particular pyscho-social aspects of care gives access to a rich description and critical evaluation of care (Box 9.1). Learning to observe and write in such a way fundamentally led me to a new way in thinking, talking and writing about patients as reflected in Johny's discharge letter.

BOX 9.1 JOHNY ARTHUR'S SPECIAL INTERVENTION SHEET

SI 1 Reflecting with Johny on his future 28/2/92

Johny said to me today – 'I don't know why you bother I've got no future'

Questions: When Johny makes such comments how do you respond?

Can we spend more time with him to show that we value him as a person?

NAME Johny Arthur PRIMARY NURSE Roger

AARON MACLEAN: A PUZZLE UNSOLVED

Using the BNDU model is not a guarantee that desired outcomes will be attained. There are some people and situations are a puzzle with no easy answers given their complexity. This is the nature of the 'messy lowlands' (Schon 1983). It is a difficult for me to admit and yet a consequence of my reflective and self-critical nature. Aaron Maclean was such a puzzle.

At the time, I felt anxious and frustrated to an extreme degree, and even now, months later reflecting on my involvement with Aaron, is scarcely more comfortable. In part this is because I have such high expectations of myself, but I do wonder how using the BNDU model may bring to the surface a practitioner's suppressed anxieties and doubts about competence. Such speculation leads me to suggest that using a holistic model requires practitioners have the necessary development to enable them to be effective. I am referring to clinical supervision. I discussed Aaron at length in clinical supervision on six occasions.

When I first talked about Aaron I noted

> *I've got a patient at the moment who is quite a puzzle to us all... with reduced mobility, chronic constipation, lethargy, low motivation, he sees no point in eating, drinking, in fact doing anything. He doesn't want to listen to people – if you persist he gets quite irritated. He requires help – two nurses to transfer him from bed to chair. He grabs people and objects. When you insist he stands better he then panics after a few minutes. I haven't had time to spend a long time with him, but I feel I have got to get down to what he wants and how to achieve that.*

Justifiably my supervisor challenged me on my statement 'I haven't had time?' I replied 'I know, I need to make time – it's bothering me.'

The question of 'making time' is one that is crucial to me in using the BNDU model in my practice. Just after one Christmas, I returned from holiday to find the hospital nearly full with very dependent people with substantial needs. Minimal assessments, mainly of physical aspects of care had been made. I wrote about this in my diary feeling depressed and angry (at the time I was the only primary nurse).

> *I meet each patient in giving them care, but was only able to plan care for essential physical requirements. I wanted to make time to reflect on the cue questions... Now – 48 hours later – I have got up-to-date with physical problems and I know I can communicate the emotional problems and needs but have not yet got these onto paper. Time is the key'. Interventions and evaluation have taken all my time but now I'll have to work on holistic assessments. Alternatively, I could have spent more of my own time to reflect on Aaron's psycho-social needs, and how these might have been better identified and met by other practitioners. But I rationalized – it does not seem a realistic sue of my time given the pressures of physical requirements – and I have maintained and promoted safety and recovery.*

As I write now, this seems more like crisis management than holistic care. Returning to Aaron, I commented to an associate nurse that I did not understand how Aaron 'worked'. In response, she admitted being baffled by him. I felt I was beginning to blame myself for this situation.

'Blame' is an interesting concept. As the primary nurse I was aware of my responsibility for Aaron's care, but I was also uneasily aware that I had crossed over the line of responsibility for my actions to take up responsibility for Aaron's actions. It was as if I believed that there was a secret key to his actions and if I engaged deeply enough with him I would find it and enable him to resolve his anxieties, take control of his physical problems and get up and go. Although not realising it at the time my involvement with Aaron had crept up on me and was beginning to consume me leaving me entangled in it! I slowly realised this was happening and I needed supervision to untangle me.

A RISKY DISCHARGE HOME – UNRESOLVED CONFLICT WITH A DISTRICT NURSE

Aaron had expressed a wish to go home. I discussed this with my colleagues and we decided that since he was not thriving in the hospital his wish should be respected. We realised it was a 'risky' discharge but that taking the risk was fully in accord with the Burford vision – 'where the patient's experience and need for control in their lives is recognized...' Therefore Aaron was entitled to the opportunity to succeed or fail at living at home with his limitations.

The hospital Occupational Therapist assessed his home resources and I discussed Aaron's wish with his GP so he would be aware of my rationale for facilitating Aaron's discharge. The GP's response was typically laconic 'If Aaron wishes that, then OK.'

I was not aware of asking the GP's permission for the discharge, and I am not sure if he interpreted it as such, but the use of 'OK' would suggest that he did so. This raises the interesting point of sharing one's work with other care workers who are not using the BNDU model. Discussing patient's wishes with their GP and conveying the GP's opinion to the patient sometimes can be a useful way of relieving anxiety. I suggested to one particular patient that she might benefit from a weekend at home but she would not consider it. I then discussed this with her GP who agreed with me that it would appear to be beneficial. When I informed her that Dr Hilary approved she replied 'well if Dr Hilary thinks it is a good idea then it must be.'

With Aaron Maclean however, his GP's opinion was marginal to our decision to follow Aaron's wish. Aaron's home carer and the district nurse were deeply sceptical but as I wrote later and shared in supervision –

> *We felt we couldn't give any more care in hospital as he wouldn't let us near him... I offered a choice to try at home for the weekend – his morale was boosted. He wanted to try. He went home where he stayed bed bound, didn't eat or drink. He was seen by Ann, the district nurse, she was distressed and angry at seeing him like that. She contacted me and feedback that sending him home was the wrong decision and that he should come back in. I agreed to this and explained that at the time I felt Aaron would benefit from the weekend to see for himself. Since he's been back he's been worse – he hasn't reflected at all on his visit home. when prompted he just changed the subject.*

My feelings were that Ann was reacting as much to her workload stress and blaming me for an inadequate discharge. She also remarked in this vein to others. I felt that her off-loading her stress clouded the issues for Aaron. I asserted my right to have my decision accepted and the validity of my viewpoint.

REFLECTION ON THE CONFLICT OF VALUES

This experience illustrates the potentially problematic position of realising a holistic vision with having to communicate with colleagues who either do not share or fully understand the meaning of a holistic vision. It led to a conflict of perception about Aaron's best interests and needs.

The issue of conflict is noted in the Burford vision,

> *That care is best given by those who care and have a respect for each other within our respective roles despite differences of opinion at times, and who can share their feelings at appropriate times openly, and who mutually support others where needed*

These words were chosen carefully to reflect the significance of the therapeutic team and allude to the difficulty which nurses have in being open to seeking and receiving feedback rather than falling back on the 'harmonious team'. My experience as a primary nurse at Burford supports Johns' (1992) findings, who suggest that assertiveness, facing conflict and sharing feelings are essential to the development of the therapeutic team. The countervailing culture of the harmonious team remains strongly resistant, like prevailing headwinds against which a cyclist might have to struggle. It is a learning curve to find time to dialogue with colleagues such as Ann to share values and make best decisions necessary to resolve conflict and meet patients' needs. What is best is always an ethical issue based on the situation as acknowledged in the model for structured reflection that Johns has constructed to guide reflection posing the cue 'Did I act for the best?' taking into the consideration of differing perspectives and ethical principles.[9]

The difficulty Ann and myself experienced over what was best for Aaron illustrated how painful conflict can be and as a consequence how defensive we both were and the need to work with each other within a therapeutic team.[10]

FOCUSING ON THE PERSON

In attempting to reach Aaron I reflected that he was a man with many barriers. I asked myself if I could see beyond these barriers. What did I mean by this? I felt that whenever I tried to offer him any care and to work with him, he responded by blocking my approaches. Even when he did not physically turn away from me he put up psychological barriers to stop me getting closer.

One morning I tried to spend the whole morning with him in an attempt to find a way out of this situation. He told me that he wanted to live, and I gave him feedback that he was killing himself by not eating and drinking. I noted that it was the first time he had answered a direct question with a direct answer. That seemed like progress and so I decided that rather than let care 'drift' along as it seemed to be doing, I had to continue to challenge him. In supervision I noted

> *On reflection I feel very frustrated – I feel I achieved very little by challenging him... this was not helped by interruptions – the telephone ringing, helping others... I had said to my colleagues that I wanted to concentrate on Aaron that morning and they agreed with that. But that didn't stop the interruptions. I could have asserted my right to stay with him rather than respond to interruptions but I learnt how difficult this work is.*

I used the Model for Structured Reflection (Appendix 2) to order my thoughts on this intervention, which helped me to understand myself better. I recognised that I wanted to widen the options of care and give my colleagues that something was being done. It also brought my feelings into sharper and painful focus.

I wrote in my journal:

> *I feel very sad and dissatisfied that I couldn't reach Aaron and feel I didn't all that I could but I don't know if it would have altered the situation... when it was happening I felt powerless and at a loss – I didn't like it at all – it made me like a bad nurse, not a good primary nurse.*

Reading through this structured reflection with my supervisor after Aaron had died helped me clarify further. The following conversation between myself (PN) and my supervisor (S):

PN: When I confronted Aaron with the consequences of his actions he either clammed up or talked about something else.
S: What did you infer from that?
PN: The impression I got was that he was very afraid of what was happening to him of losing control and dying. He couldn't admit it to me. I challenged him with the contradiction but he didn't respond.
S: Perhaps you were getting too close?
PN: I feel I ought to have known what to do.
S: That sounds like the medical model?
PN: It does in a way... I didn't see it that way at the time... I just wanted to help him and I couldn't.

POSTSCRIPT

I began Aaron's case study with the statement that the holistic model is not a guarantee in itself that desired outcomes will be attained, but I feel that this in no way invalidates the model. Rather it suggests to me that the model is a powerful motivation for the practitioner to persist with rather than be wholly discouraged by problematic situations. My experience with Aaron suggests that it would have been more painful without the challenge, support and valid feedback of clinical supervision. I left the supervision session still feeling unhappy. I did not feel that 40 minutes talking had eased my distress. However, cycling home along country roads I felt a little better. The next morning, the first day of my substantial holiday in the six and a half months since becoming a primary nurse at Burford, I woke up feeling much happier and reckoned that my reflections had enabled me to come to terms with myself. In my next supervision session I reported

> *Next morning I woke up and felt a great weight had lifted from me – that I hadn't picked up, and had been harder on myself than I needed to have been. It was like a delayed benefit from the session.*

Reflections on using the BNDU model compared with using other models in previous experience

A year after I began using the BNDU model I feel as if I am still scratching the surface of its potential. But compared with my previous application of nursing models I retain my initial excitement and intuition that there is further potential in me to realise my holistic beliefs about nursing in practice. What do I mean by this?

Simply, that there is something underneath the superficial structure of the model. It seems to have the potential to open the way to dealing with psychosocial aspects of care in a profound way. Sometimes I feel I have never listened to patients before, and I hear such a wealth of information and insights that I cannot set it all down. Yet, what may appear to be a chance or passing remark provides me with invaluable insights into peoples' lives, how they are feeling and how they view themselves and regarding the future.

Previously I had used the familiar yet bland cues of the Roper, Logan and Tierney model with the activities of living and life span continuum. When I wish to define specific physical activities, such as a mobility plan of care or wound, this model would be adequate but limiting. Most practitioners will prescribe actions and interventions with which they are familiar. Of course, this is natural not to challenge themselves to look beyond their normal practice or horizons. The BNDU model, by contrast, lends to such a widening of possibility. For example, in approaching the care of an extremely anxious man I outlined what he had told me, describing the ways I had observed his anxiety and asked my colleagues to do likewise to –

> *consider the strategies which might help [this person] to allay his anxieties, and, from interactions, note strategies which appear helpful or unhelpful.*

I am prepared to admit that I do not know all the approaches that might be therapeutic, and I see my colleagues, my patients, and their carers as collaborators with me rather than slaves to my care plan or passive objects of care. It is clear, that as a primary nurse I am responsible for initiating plans of care for my patients, but if either patients, carers, or colleagues at any time find these inappropriate or inadequate they are encouraged to challenge or alter my plan provided they can offer a valid rationale.

Accountability relates to our belief at Burford that a primary nurse needs to grasp and explore the personal boundaries of autonomy, that is

> *the freedom to make decisions within the boundaries of defined practice together with the freedom to act on those decisions. (Johns 1990:886)*

At Burford this autonomy is balanced with collaboration –

> *of a therapeutic team that actively encourages and supports its members to explore and share their work. (Johns 1990:889)*

These are attractive words, but in reality it is difficult to achieve because, as qualified nurses, we are acculturated to the harmonious team, which sees conflict and the giving and receiving of valid but potentially uncomfortable feedback as too painful. I find it easier to avoid conflict, but I also know that such evasion often prevents or delays outcomes that my patients, colleagues and I see as desirable. Avoidance does not permit resolution of conflict but suppresses and fuels it. The outcomes of care within the framework of the BNDU model can be measured through developing standards of care, a process of group critical reflection focusing on discrete aspects of practice. By doing this we –

> *Publically demonstrate that the actions of nurses makes a qualitatively difference to peoples' lives. (Johns 1991:1095)*

However, it is in the field of day-to-day relationships with colleagues, that escaping from the old ideas is hard, and the application of new ones equally so. In other environments of care I have felt constrained by a rigid vertical hierarchy and an uneasy combination of biological systems model within a dominant medical model. To repeat myself, psychological care was largely unplanned or defined superficially if recognised at all with such expression as 'give the patient time to ask questions and express anxieties' or the ubiquitous 'give reassurance' as if some lip service to the notion. Patients' profound psychological and spiritual needs were addressed at time but I suspect this was despite the nursing model not because of it.

The Burford model has emerged out of practice and returns to practice for testing and increasing sophistication (Johns 1991:1097). Through the cue questions and the special intervention sheets I am able to explore my caring potential and reach towards realising our collective vision of holistic practice. It is in my hands as a clinical practitioner.

My engagement with the BNDU model has been a long adventurous journey – an odyssey. My understanding of and value for the model has deepened. Writing this account contributes to its validation alongside others' accounts beyond mere anecdote, because of how I have become critically reflective of the model as a natural part of my everyday practice, testing it without necessarily realising I was testing it for its validity to frame and facilitate holistic practice as intended through its vision.

It is of particular pertinence that I have had this opportunity to reflect on my engagement with the BNDU model because we are preparing for a critical review of the vision, an event I am eagerly anticipating. It seems a paradox that I feel attuned to the model, and the model fits the practice I aspire to, but I do not feel attuned to the vision. This is not because I have profound disagreement with it but welcome the opportunity to contribute and owning the vision rather than just signing up to it.

NOTES

1 Initially I termed guided reflection sessions 'professional supervision'.

2 Sachs's words say much about the nature of holistic practice. Roger illustrates how extant ideas from whatever source are inspirational and help to frame something that may seem intangible.

3 Roger illuminates that using the Burford model is not simply replacing one model (Roper, Logan and Tierney) with another. It is more profound than that – holistic nursing is a new mindset where old norms no longer work. He wants to fill in boxes. He wants structure. Give me physical problems. He is used to that way of approaching practice. Give someone too much freedom and he can drown. In his journal he reflects that he thought he was reflective before but now realises that reflection goes much deeper to become an intrinsic part of practice.

4 These were monthly meetings between primary and associate nurses without my 'leadership' presence held alternatively at the hospital and a social setting to strengthen the therapeutic team.

5 Roger's 'Who am I?' was hidden in his previous work. As such using the model is cathartic as evidenced in Roger's account. It follows that shifting to the Burford NDU model requires significant challenge and support requiring systems as guided reflection and the therapeutic team – yet as Roger highlights, the therapeutic team requires another fundamental shift in nursing culture. His colleagues were able to confront and support him and deal positively with conflict.

6 A shift in culture requires a different attitude towards doctors. Roger illustrates his 'winging' to the GP as seeking some permission not to care for Madge and also permission to send a patient home for weekend visit. To what extent Roger was able to break free from perceiving himself in a subordinate role is not easy to ascertain – yet he was aware of his role and relationship vis-a-vis doctors was an issues to reflect on.

7 Let's face it. Every practice will have difficulties with attitudes to patients who are very dependent and non-cooperative. Madge was initially seen through a lens of workload and

lack of resources to care for her adequately. Yet that was an illusion – as Roger indicated with right attitude and resources. Limitations are only in the mind. What was profound, was that once Roger and his colleagues had broken through their initial limited perception of Madge she was a joy to care for.

8 Reflexive narrative was developed as the means for written communication and continuity of care (see Chapter 4). Narrative reflects the person's journey through their health-illness experience prompted by the continuous assessment and evaluation through using the Burford NDU model cues. The traditional paucity of written notes reflects the oral tradition in nursing and the essential intuitive nature of emotional care. Understanding these issues led to the development of *Special Intervention* sheets as a more expressive way to communicate psychosocial aspects of care, pulling out these issues from the general narrative.

9 'Did I act for the best?' is a cue within the Model for structured reflection (see Appendix 3).

10 Arranging this discharge created conflict with the district nurse that highlights the potential difficulty of using the Burford model in association with others who do not share the Burford vision. Hence the idea of holism was a threat to the district nurse because it disrupted her normal view of patients. It shows the need for a deeper collaboration where perspectives can be explored through dialogue leading to an understanding and including the district nurse into the therapeutic team crossing boundaries of care. Perhaps then Roger's actions will influence and shift the district nurse's perspective. As such Roger becomes an advocate for the vision in being an advocate for the patient.

REFERENCES

Johns C (1990) Autonomy of primary nurses: the need to both facilitate and limit autonomy in practice. *Journal of Advanced Nursing* 15; 886–94.

Johns C (1991) The Burford nursing development unit holistic model for nursing practice. *Journal of Advanced Nursing* 16; 1090–8.

Johns C (1992) Ownership and the harmonious team: barriers to developing the therapeutic nursing team in primary nursing. *Journal of Clinical Nursing* 1; 89–94.

Sacks O (1990) *Awakenings* (revised edition) Picador, London.

Schon D (1983) *The reflective practitioner: how professionals think in action*. Basic Books, New York.

Just Following Care? Reflections of Associate Nurses in Using the BNDU Model at Burford

CHAPTER 10

Kate Butcher and Jan Dewing

In this chapter we reflect on our experience with the BNDU model from the perspectives of our associate nurse roles at Burford. This account reflects our personal involvement in practice using the model.

THE ROLE OF THE ASSOCIATE NURSE

Our roles, as associate nurses, are very different. Kate is employed as an associate nurse. Jan works as an associate nurse within her role as hospital manager and lecturer-practitioner. We therefore bring different perspectives, knowledge and skills to our mutual roles.

The role of the associate nurse is essentially to follow the prescribed care planned by the primary nurse and to respond to changing circumstances in the absence of the primary nurse as appropriate (Manthey 1980). In fulfilling this role, the BNDU model gives us 'artistic licence' to be the nurses we are, and strive towards the nurses we hope to become. In other words, we are practitioners in our own right with beliefs and feelings that are important determinants in the care we give.[1]

From the perspective of a lecturer-practitioner my clinical work can either be planned and given over several spans of duty so I can practice nursing for myself or as a role model for other staff or it may be on an occasional span 'here and there' to fill in gaps for whatever reason. I need to be able to nurse in a clinical role for myself because I am a nurse. I need to have relationships with patients, relatives, nurses and other clinical staff because it provides a source of motivation and questioning for me to carry out aspects of my role in education and management.

Because I know I am working with patients and colleagues for a limited period of time I want to work as intensely and effectively as I can to maximise my contribution to patient care. I would argue that in both instances, but especially 'here and now', the written communication generated by the BNDU model enables me to gain a clear insight of the patient's

Holistic Practice in Healthcare: The Burford NDU Person-centred Model, Second Edition. Edited by Christopher Johns.

perception of the meaning of their illness, together with the feelings and ideas of the primary nurses who had planned care. This enables me to feel more part of the nursing team and that care for the patients has more continuity and consistency even delivered by such a part time nurse.

However, from the perspective of associate nurses who may be part-time, or newly qualified, or returning from practice following a break, using the BNDU model may be more challenging. These nurses may be lacking in confidence. To get the best out of the model requires nurses to be creative and this often means taking risks and exposing themselves. This requires an enabling type of leadership.

PERSONAL PHILOSOPHIES

The starting point to working creatively with the BNDU model is to examine one's personal philosophy of nursing. We both share many similarities in our personal philosophies, yet in many ways they are very different. That we do share many similarities is reassuring; as this is necessary in order to offer patients consistent and congruent care (Johns 1991). Perhaps the main reason they are different is that they are never complete and hence are at different stages of their conception as would be expected considering our diverse backgrounds and experience.

Our personal philosophies are reflected in the hospital's written philosophy. As such, we own it. It has meaning for us unlike other models we have experienced that merely reflect the author's view of how nursing should be often wrapped up in an obscure language that makes little practical sense.

Reflecting on our experiences often highlights contradictions between our beliefs and values and the way we practice, given us insight to work at resolving these contradictions in practice and future reflection. In doing so we test and clarify our visions of practice. Hence the BNDU philosophy has real practical intent.

KATE'S EXPERIENCE USING THE BNDU MODEL

The following case studies all aim to illustrate my understanding and use of the BNDU in practice. Reflection on these studies in supervision facilitated my learning and development as a nurse.

JACK AND SARAH

In this first case study I progressed from working alongside the primary nurse to becoming the primary nurse following the primary nurse's resignation. At this point I had been qualified just 8 weeks.

Jack Roberts was admitted to Burford, accompanied by his wife Sarah, following a collapse in his garden. He was a retired naval officer, 'a gentleman' as his GP described him. Now he was aphasic with a dense right-sided weakness. Sarah was distraught especially due to the fact they had only married two years previously.

Along with planning Jack's care following a diagnosis of cerebral vascular accident, care was also offered to Sarah. This is integral due to our assessment question 'who is this person?' that necessitates a holistic assessment which naturally extends to the family. Since Sarah was Jack's support in life – this is linked to the cue question 'what support does this person have in life?' – it was natural that Sarah's needs were considered. A Special intervention sheet [SI] was developed headed 'Counselling Mrs. Roberts', upon which were recorded relevant comments and conversations from Sarah which indicated her level of coping. The primary nurse had spoken with Sarah on a number of occasions so that when I took responsibility for Jack's care I found the recorded notes of considerable value. Comments such as – 'it's a complete reversal of role. Jack was always the strong partner' and 'It's the lack of communication I can't deal with, we used to talk so much' were recorded along with information such as Sarah's wish that Jack should be discharged to a nursing home rather than go home on completion of his care at Burford. She also explained how difficult she found helping Jack to wash and dress despite wanting to help. Such recorded information helped me to validate her actions such as unexpected hesitancy and shyness when I became responsible for their care.

This case study illustrates the holism of the BNDU model in that care was extended to include the family of the patient, which, in my limited experience is an often neglected issues of care as partners are seen as individuals in their own right, but less often as an integral part of the individual requiring care. Sarah and Jack were a couple very much involved in each other's lives. Therefore to care for Jack we had to care for Sarah. This meant offering Sarah care that she would have expected from jack had he been able to give it, for example, emotional support since Jack could not talk.

Another significant cue was 'how do they view the future for themselves and others?' Since Jack could not tell us, we had to ask Sarah, and it was then that we discovered not only Sarah's wish for a nursing home but also the stress she was experiencing which we could help to alleviate. Since the cue questions are precisely that, a cue, a prompt to aid thinking, each cue does not require an answer but the ones I have noted proved themselves to be invaluable in planning Jack's care. Without these I imagine that care offered to Sarah would have been inconsistent between different staff members and that Jack's future may not have been considered with as much individualisation as it was.

The use of the model eased my transition from being an associate nurse to becoming a primary nurse for this family in that all the information I initially needed was provided through the notes. I had only to make myself better known to all those involved and adapt to the altered responsibility. Thanks to the BNDU model I felt that I had already begun to 'know' the family and felt that the care I could offer would be individualised. I had never before felt this when reading notes written based on other models. However, had my practical experience been greater I may have been more able to enhance the care we offered Sarah, rather than merely following the plan already set.

The model allows for a considerable degree of creativity on the part of each nurse involved in its use, but to achieve this, experience and confidence are necessary. I do not feel that we offered Jack and Sarah a poor standard of care but acknowledge through reflection that we may have improved their care. The extent that I was able to be therapeutic with Jack and Sarah depended very much at the time on my degree of experience, and I felt quite strongly at this point that a nurse with greater experience than myself may have worked differently (low self-esteem eight weeks after qualifying as a nurse placed a voice in my head saying 'better' rather than 'differently').

However, the BNDU model focuses on each nurse's areas for development due to its reflective nature, and thus turns each experience into a learning situation. Therefore, although I had some negative feelings I still felt supported by the model since I felt that any nurse, regardless of any amount of experience would have learnt something and so I was not alone. Undoubtedly, dialogue and feedback with my supervisor was a significant asset to challenge and support me, affirming my work and boosting my fragile self-esteem.

MILDRED

This second case study illustrates my change role to a 'trainee' primary nurse, that is, acting as a primary nurse to one patient with support from other staff members.

Mildred Baker was admitted for rehabilitation following a fall on ice when she sustained fractures of the humerus and tibia. She also suffered from multiple health problems including polymyalgia and diverticulitis. She had a close and loving family who visited regularly, and a strong religious faith, both of which provided her support for life.

I wrote in my assessment that she –

> *relies heavily on the fact that she can be of help to others and consequently feels useless' at being in hospital unable to physically help herself, never mind others, and that 'she feels she no longer has her health.*

Due to the fractures and her prevailing chronic conditions that were quite obviously incorporated into an already adjusted health condition. Now Mildred had to temporarily adjust further to her fractures. My comments acknowledged, and maybe even predicted, Mildred's lack of coping mechanisms to deal with her situation and allowed me to plan for such.

Three weeks later when writing her narrative I noted

> *Although her physiotherapy is progressing well, Mildred does not seem to believe in this, or have faith in herself, relying more and more on our reassurance.*

Continuing assessment within the narrative form is demanded of the BNDU model as we develop a greater understanding of the person and develop trusting relationships enabling deeper insight into their situation, and because a person's state of health often fluctuates, as in the case of Mildred. As her primary nurse, I was responsible for Mildred's continuous assessment and evaluation of Mildred's care, and as noted previously with Jack and Sarah's care, I found the assessment cues invaluable especially with regard to psychosocial aspects of care – the cues 'who is this person?' and 'what support does this person have in life?'

However, writing her care plan in response to these cues was not easy as whatever I wrote seemed to patronise and stereotype. For example –

Mildred is anxious due to hospital admission

Goal – to reassure

Action – give Mildred time to talk about her feelings

Such documentation made me feel as though the care I would then be giving was not individualised because I had written such words many times previously as a student and read it so many times too. To overcome this feeling I found it useful to use a 'Special Intervention' sheet to record her increased dependence for support upon staff rather than her getting this from her family or faith as she had done on admission.

I wrote how I thought staff should approach Mildred in a suggestive rather than prescriptive manner that acknowledged my colleagues might have approaches that were equally valid or more so. This was important to me as I felt as a student that I was only performing a set of functions that someone else thought appropriate where my own individuality and thoughts could not show through the care. This attitude made me feel devalued and mindful of that, I did not want my colleagues to feel the same way in their care of Mildred.

'Special Intervention' sheets demand creativity because they are blank sheets of paper. They can be both empowering and stressful. The empowerment arises from an acknowledgment of the nurse's skill at developing holistic care, the freedom to be creative within collective beliefs, and the chance to work as a team in fulfilling the challenge set out on the sheet. However, stress can quickly arise from this freedom, the stress of 'not knowing' the best action to take because the situation has not been encountered previously, of feeling inexperienced and incompetent. This last point is highlighted through the freedom of the assessment tool. Whereas, for example, Roper et al.'s model (used as a comparison because this was the model I encountered on each ward I worked on as a student) would expect some perspective on the physical aspects of care such as elimination or breathing, the BNDU model poses a vague question (as I interpreted it since it did not direct me to think of specific activities of living) 'what health event brings this person into hospital?' For someone like me, a recently qualified practitioner as I was at the time (approximately 4 months) this did not guide me to think about problems such as constipation due to diverticulitis.[2]

Whilst I acknowledge that the reason behind such omission was my own inexperience, the model was not quite the guide I had hoped for, therefore making the situation more stressful. Whilst I am not suggesting that other models excuse practitioners from thinking for themselves, they may focus or direct the thoughts more quickly thus seeming less stressful at the time. On reflection, I now view that more directive models could be seen as restrictive if not used to their full potential, for example the Roper et al.'s model is often interpreted as only being a list of 12 activities of living, and I consider the BNDU model is liberating in its use.

I found the cue – 'How does this person make me feel?' to be of incredible value during Mildred's stay as I found my relationship with her changing throughout her stay. I discussed the situation in my supervision – '*As Mildred gets to know me I feel that she is manipulating me.*'

In terms of being therapeutic, having access to such feelings was invaluable since I was able to recognise the reasoning behind my actions, for example, becoming more detached from Mildred. Through reflection, I was able to identify the effect upon Mildred of this withdrawal and also predict how I could cope with my feelings more effectively, to become more poised to be more available to her.

The BNDU model, being reflective in nature by asking 'How does this person make me feel?' put me into contact with my own feelings more than I had ever been and so enabled me to act positively to overcome my negative feelings such as manipulation. This was a big issue for me in caring for Mildred as I felt we were moving away from working in partnership with one another with Mildred being 'in charge'. This seems paradoxical as my aim was ultimately for Mildred to be in control of her situation, but through her manner she was not making informed choices and therefore I felt I was battling against her. Had we remained in the 'partnership' state I could have offered advice more comfortably and so prevented my stress.

This case study indicates that students and newly qualified staff may struggle to use the BNDU model because of its lack of structure without strong guidance, peer support, and gaining experience in the associate nurse role before assuming primary nurse responsibility. It also highlights how previous acculturation to one particular model can make it difficult to using a different, less prescriptive, kind of model based on reflection and thinking.

BERT

In this description of Bert's admission to Burford I assumed the most commonly portrayed role of the associate nurse, that of following the care as planned by the primary nurse and reporting any changes needed for their approval (Pearson 1988, Manthey 1980).

Bert Johnson was an intelligent and articulate man, widely travelled and very knowledgeable. He was admitted to Burford for respite care on a regular basis. He had worsening emphysema and was reliant on oxygen therapy. He was interested in the idea of individualised care and assisted the primary nurse in the development of his care plan. During the admission Bert identified the problem 'I am unable to spend my days at Burford as I would do at home'. With the underlying current of now being unable to live his life as he was used to due to his illness that restricted his activities.

During each previous admission, Bert seemed to enjoy making staff feel uncomfortable by humiliating them due to their lack of knowledge, for example he would order his lunch in Dutch. Because of this, staff would try to have minimal contact with him due to the unpleasant feelings his behaviour created. For this reason, there were areas of his assessment not completed as comprehensively as they could have been.

Bert Johnson's admission occurred during a quiet period of work giving me more time to get to know Bert more intimately, and to dispel the preconceptions I had gathered from other staff. I did this ostensibly for my own reasons – Bert made me feel uncomfortable and I wanted to put an end to this. Whenever I had 'free' time I would sit with Bert, allowing him to lead the conversation. I found that by giving him some of my attention when he knew I could be elsewhere he became less demanding and critical, grateful for my honesty, for example when I said 'This is interesting but can we continue it later when I have more time to spend with you.' He also became more open with himself, speaking of his feelings and anxieties relating to his deteriorating condition.

I discussed my 'breakthrough' with Bert's primary nurse and write a SI sheet

> *On talking with Bert I have found him to be a pleasant and interesting and considerate man. He knows how he is perceived by others – a moaner, demanding, boring, a miserable old man – but also expresses feelings of loneliness and a fear of his deteriorating condition and eventual death. I feel we have not been aware of this situation and responded to him a little brusquely. As such, I challenge our attitude towards him (including my own) and suggest we spend time with him when we can. He does understand that we have other people to care for and only expects politeness and honesty.*

The prompts for me writing about my experience in this way were the cue questions 'Who is this person?' and 'How does this person make me feel?' and subsequently 'How is this person feeling?' and 'what is important to make his stay in hospital comfortable?' Whilst these cues had been considered by the primary nurse, we had different perceptions highlighting the subjective nature of the cues and hence perception of the person. It emphasised the need to dialogue between staff to find mutual understanding to ensure a coherent approach to care.

The cue question 'How does this person make me feel?' prompted me to access and deal with my feelings, enabling me to confront my negative attitude and hence become more available to work therapeutically with Bert. This was of great importance to me as many other staff members had rejected him.

In supervision I reflected on my relationship with Bert using Transactional Analysis (Berne 1964). I recognised that Bert had been treating me like 'child' and humiliating me with his language. At first I responded as 'hurt child', but worked through that rejecting this ego state to respond as an 'adult' – creating our difficulty with communication. According to Berne's theory, in any interaction we can adopt one of three roles: parent, adult and child. Clear lines of communication exist between like or opposite roles but difficulties occur when lines are crossed such as between adult and child.

Once a relationship of honesty had been established with Bert we were able to relate to each other either as 'adult-adult' or 'parent-child'. If Bert reverted to his humiliation tactics I was able to respond positively by shifting myself into the child role of accepting the 'parent's' teaching, thus saving myself from humiliation and protecting Bert from my ensuing anger.[3]

KEY POINTS

1. The interpretation of the cue questions; i.e. their subjective nature
2. The development of therapeutic relationships (one where both Bert and myself received positive feelings)
3. The notion of holism prompted by 'who is this person?' and involving Bert in his care planning
4. The link between the assessment cues (one leading to another)
5. The use of Special Intervention sheets to communicate willing all staff to develop a more positive relationship with Bert (and in the process confronting negative attitudes towards him)

DEVELOPING MY EXPERTISE

From these three case studies I have illustrated how experience and confidence affect the use of the BNDU model. Whilst it was of value in the first case study, as a newly qualified practitioner I lacked confidence to expand upon it. Following the primary nurse's care plan was easy due to her thoroughness, inexperience inhibited me from developing it further which, perhaps I could have done using a familiar model such as the Roper, Logan and Tierney model with which I was acquainted.

In the second case study my confidence and experience had grown to the extent I could assess a person reasonably well. However, I felt the BNDU model blinded me from considering a more subtle aspect of physical care I would probably have noted if following the Roper et al. model. In my final case study with Bert, I am much more confident and begin to use the BNDU model creatively, to the point I am able to consider my influence upon an individual and vice versa and thus the model leads me to a much more therapeutic care.

JAN'S EXPERIENCE

The following case study describes my admission assessment in the absence of the primary nurse. In many senses this was a 'holiday activity' by me in my associate nurse role, yet it provided much valuable information for the primary nurse 'to pick up' who used it as a basis for developing her relationship with the patient rather than repeating the assessment.[4]

JOAN

Joan was a 67-year-old woman who came to the hospital for assessment following a request from her GP. The day before her admission she reported a sudden loss of function in her legs. There did not appear to be any apparent reason for this. The history given to the GP was unclear as both Joan and her family were very panicked by what was happening. Joana's sister and daughter had looked after her on the sofa overnight.

Very quickly, during talking to Joan, I could see that it was not appropriate to carry out a full assessment. Joan was very tired, she had little sleep the night before and she was anxious about being in hospital. She got into bed with all her clothes on, even her coat, and declined to remove them for several hours.

Despite being very conscious of my interviewing skills Joan gave very short factual responses to my questions. She was unable to answer questions that were open-ended and those that related to how she felt about what was happening. She sat very still in the bed and did not respond. Her eye contact with me, despite my seating and body positioning, was minimal.

During an assessment I am always pleased if I gain insight into the person and their perception of their health. I regard assessments as an on-going process, like a jigsaw, and think the initial assessment should be as non-invasive as possible. The BNDU model reflects this shared belief that the assessment should be sensitive and on-invasive. For Joan, it was not appropriate to continue with a detailed assessment. It was even possible that she did not want to talk at all. Following the interview I began to reflect on why I thought this way using the cue questions below–

'HOW DOES THE PATIENT MAKE ME FEEL?'

I felt hat Joan was not interested in talking with me, but I was able to understand that this was not personal. Had I thought that, I might not have gone back to her or questioned myself any further about what was happening. I realised I was reading her body language and her verbal and non-verbal cues which were indicating to me that she was not interested in talking.

It seemed to me that Joan's face had a mask expression almost as if she was unresponsive or devoid of emotion. Her voice was flat and expressionless. I began to consider that she may be like this because she was frightened or that the loss of functioning had affected her non-verbal and verbal communication skills or that she poorly skilled in communicating her feelings. I also considered that she may have another pathological problem which we did not know about such as Parkinson's disease, or that she was taking medications that caused her to appear uncreative or devoid of emotion. I had also noticed the way in which her family assisted her to settle into bed. I observed them relating to her almost as if she was a child. They talked to her using simple language with a lot of instructions and Joan did not always respond to them. Although I thought that their behaviour could be a reflection of their anxiety, it seemed to be deeper than this.

I needed to consider the next cue question.

'HOW CAN I BEST HELP THIS PERSON?'

When I shared my feelings of uncertainty about not knowing how best to help Joan at this time because I could not work out what she wanted and because she could not communicate with me clearly, the daughter and sister immediately knew what I meant. They told me it was the effect of the medication she was taking and that she could not help it. I asked them how they thought she was feeling. They told me things that Joan said and how she behaved when anxious. They said Joan needed lots of reassurance and affection. They also said she did not seem to acknowledge it, but she did appreciate it. This then added another dimension to my assessment of Joan, leading to the next cue.

'HOW IS THIS PERSON FEELING?'

After reflecting on this new information, I was able to think that Joan might not be feeling as calm or detached as she appeared. Her sister and daughter described to me how Joan switched off completely when she was worried about something. I knew now that she was not uncreative or devoid of emotion, but I had thought that she had wanted to be on her own, and wondered if she would be unable to ask for help and was therefore feeling very isolated. Perhaps she had perceived my behaviour as showing little concern for her because I had not shown her affection.

From a distance I observed her resting in bed and her sleep pattern such as her movements and breathing. When I judged that she was no longer asleep but lying with her eyes closed I went and sat beside her and quietly said 'when you feel like opening your eyes I will help you do what you want to do'. After a few minutes she opened her eyes and said 'I need to use the toilet but I don't know if I can.' When she said this her face was still expressionless as was her voice.

I knew that for Joan it was becoming very frightening because she was losing her functions very quickly; it seemed to her that every time she tried to do something else she lost the ability. She was perplexed and could not make sense what was happening to her. She needed help but felt cut off from other people because of the way she presented herself and the way other people interpreted their first impressions of her.

Because I stopped and reflected on the events surrounding Joan's admission using the cue questions flexibly I was able to see how the situation might be from Joan's perspective. This insight then influenced the direction of care I was able to give and the information I gave the nurse coming on for night duty.

USING THE ASSESSMENT CUES

The cue questions form an adaptable framework for practice. As Salvage (1990) states – nursing models open up new channels of communication and provide a fresh focus of work interest for the benefit of nurses as well as patients. When primary nurses are handing over their patients to us, we know they are using information gleaned from the cue questions as the basis for their impression and planned care of the patient. Hence we are on the same wavelength enabling mutual understanding and continuation of care.

As associate nurses we add to the patient narrative prompted the internalised cues never accepting the planned care as it stands on face value, but always critically reflecting on its validity to support practice as we find it. As with Joan, who she is as a person develops nuances as we get to know her over time, not simply as we perceived her on admission.

The cues are just that cues, not requiring them to be actually spoken. With some patients it may be appropriate to use the cues as questions, but with most patients this has not been appropriate. This gives us freedom to work with patients using any strategies we have. When we collect and reflect on the information gained we then use the cues to form a framework.

DOROTHY

The following information could be a standard nursing entry in the patient's notes following a span of duty. The patient is a woman of 97 years of age. She has been admitted for treatment of an infection. During her admission she was confused and expressed paranoid ideas. She declared she wanted to be left to die. The GP documented that her wishes should be respected. The nurse wrote:

> *The patient has been very demanding and difficult, and aggressive to staff. She is confused and disorientated. She has constantly been shouting and swearing. She has refused any care and refused all fluids.*

This entry is reflective of a de-personalised approach by the nurse. The patient has no name. She is described as being demanding and difficult by the nurse because she does not accept the care that is on offer. The nurse is not able to form a relationship with the patient and cannot use any helpful strategies, so rather than identify this weakness in her practice the nurse projects her discomfort onto the patient. The nurse justifies her inability to care for the patient by stating the patient is confused and disorientated. These two terms are often used together and inappropriately by nurses. Because it is assumed that the patient is not to be actively treated, the nurse does not question the doctor's assessment of the patient's wishes and accordingly prescribes a low priority to trying to work therapeutically with the patient.

A contrasting entry written following the BNDU cues as a framework might look something like this:

> *Dorothy has been distressed this morning. She is not as disorientated as she was last night. She appears confused. She makes reference to God punishing her by sending thunder and lightning. However, I feel from Dorothy's perspective that makes sense. The lightning was the bright morning sun shining on her face. The tree obscured the sun intermittingly and it suddenly hit her in the eyes. In view of her poor vision the effect of the light seems like lightning. The thunder is probably the main door opening and closing. Her foments about the thunder correlate with someone opening and closing the door. I have attended to these things and Dorothy is not so distressed.*
>
> *Dorothy continues to believe that I am trying to poison her and strikes out if I offer her any water. She is very thirsty and states that she is dying for a drink but cannot take it. I have arranged for her friends to bring in some water and her favourite foods to see if she will take it from them. I have found that the most useful way to help Dorothy is to spend a few minutes with her and then she will take sips of water. If I spend more than a few minutes she becomes distressed and agitated by my presence and refused water.*
>
> *I am trying to find ways of getting her to eat and drink. But I am finding it very frustrating. I believe she wants to drink but thinks she is being poisoned. I do not believe that Dorothy is ready to die. I feel she has a mental health problem which prevents her from helping herself. It is this I find the most difficult as it is blocking Dorothy from accepting our help.*

This case study intends to highlight several key points in using the BNDU model:

1. It shows the nurse attempting to view the situation from the person's perspective notably of trying to make sense of Dorothy's reference to thunder and lightning.
2. It shows use of several cues – these include considering how the patient is feeling, how best to help the patient, and how the patient is making the nurse feel.

3. The helping strategies the nurse is trying to work out are small ones, such as ways of getting Dorothy to drink. But it shows that this is still important as it is often the smaller aspects of caring for patients that get left out of the nursing records and nursing discussions.
4. It shows the importance that these aspects of care are acknowledged so that they can be learnt by other nurses.
5. It shows that the nurse recognises the need to make positive use of support Dorothy has from her friends.
6. It shows how the nurse is considering how the patient is affecting her and how she feels about her care and about the patient. The nurse recognises that she feels frustrated by not being able to help Dorothy in the way she intended to, but does not blame Dorothy for that or try to cover up her inability to help Dorothy.[5]

BOB

The following conversation occurred between myself (the associate nurse AN) and Bob (a patient) after helping him to the toilet. Following his lunch he had been incontinent of faeces and had needed to be cleaned and have his clothing changed.

BOB: 'Are you the cook?'
AN: 'No. Is there something you would like to tell the cook?'
BOB: 'No' (pause)
AN: 'Do you think the cook would be doing what I have just done?'
BOB: 'Who are you then?' .... 'A nurse?'
AN: 'Yes... is that a surprise?'
BOB: 'God save us! Why can't you do your job properly!'
AN: 'What should I have done? Please tell me.'
BOB: 'What you're paid for. Standing around doing nothing. Worse than useless. You should be helping me rather than making me do things.'
AN: 'So what have I done? What was undressing you, washing you, dressing you and helping you walk back to here meant to be?'
BOB: 'If you can call that help.'
AN: 'How would you like us to help you?'
BOB: 'Do your job properly. Are you satisfied with what you do? You make a poor Nurse.'
AN: 'I'm finding it difficult to know how to help you because you're not treating me as an equal. We can only help you if you let us. You have to want us to help you.'
BOB: 'It seems to me that you keep everyone alive as long as you can so they suffer and you do as little as you can.'
AN: 'I can understand that it may seem like that to you. Many of the patients here, although they are disabled and unwell, may not feel like you... do you feel you are suffering?'
BOB: 'I you're going to lecture me you can clear off.'

Prior to this conversation Bob had never entered into any conversation with any of the nurses. We had this feeling that he was angry about having a stroke and he resenetd the way it disabled him. We also felt that he did not value what the nurses were trying to help him. He dismissed our care and yet declined to enter into any partnership to work out something better for himself. He even declined to negotiate partnership of any kind with his primary nurse.

In this conversation these views are confirmed. By reflecting-in-action I recognised that I had the opportunity to establish a dialogue with Bob because of the way in which he spoke and of preceding events. I tried to work out, as the conversation progressed, what Bob was feeling, how I could best find out more about who this person was and how I could best help him. I recognised that Bob was trying to devalue me and my help because he felt angry with himself needing help. I had to get beyond this in order to achieve a therapeutic interaction with him. I also let Bob see that the nurses wanted to work with him, conforming and supporting the work done by his primary nurse. It would have been easy to have risen to the insults Bob gave out.

Although Bob ended the conversation when it became too close to him, some valuable insights into how Bob was feeling about himself and how he felt about his future and his nursing care was gained. I also felt it was appropriate for Bob to end the conversation in his way so that he felt he still had some control over his situation.

On reflection, I can identify ways in which I could have tried to facilitate the conversation to develop further, so I realise that this was not a 'textbook example of communication skills', but it is important to provide real examples of what happens and how the BNDU model is used as a dynamic framework for practice.

USE OF SPECIAL INTERVENTION SHEETS [SI]

Using SIs enable practitioners to be creative. They can be used in many ways to increase nurses' awareness about aspects of care that are difficult to factually document in a care plan, such as working out the most useful way to help a patient cope positively with their anxiety or as a means of giving detailed planning for an aspect of health education or patient teaching.[6]

MRS. LAMPETER

For example, when devising an aromatherapy plan for Mrs. Lampeter we were able to use the SI based around using massage with essential oils to help her feel more positive about recovery. The primary nurse was keen on the idea and asked if something could be worked out. This demonstrates the confidence of the primary nurse: although she did not have the knowledge and skills, she enabled the associate nurse to utilise her skills and demonstrated her willingness to be taught basic massage techniques by the associate nurse. Mrs. Lampeter described her problems as sickness, aching in the legs, pain in the abdomen and not being able to sleep.

The SI listed these problems and the blend and concentration of essential oils to use in a leg massage. It also showed how the oils were tested on Mrs. Lampeter for sensitivity, and how and when the massage should be carried out.[7]

LARRY

Larry had Parkinson's disease and came in for respite care started to have hallucinations. The day before, he had increased his medication and I assessed that his disturbed behaviour was probably due to toxicity from the medication. The GP prescribed a major tranquilliser should the nurses feel it should be given.

I needed to reflect on how I felt about working with Larry when he was hallucinating and how Larry was feeling. I had to do this first before working out how I could best help Larry. I needed to be sure that I had no fear of working with Larry and that I could identify therapeutic interventions for helping him. I assessed that he was not a danger to himself and that he was safe in the hospital environment.

I decided that although I could give a low priority to Larry, in effect to leave him to get on with it and only intervene when there was a problem, this was not the best way of helping him. Neither did I want to use the tranquillisers as this would only have been to make his behaviour easier for me to manage. I decided to spend time with Larry to see if I could help him but mindful at the same time that my presence might actually disturb him.

As it was Larry was not disturbed by my presence and that he seemed to seek out companionship. He talked about what he felt was happening to him. From this, I realised that he had some insight into the hallucinations and could be facilitated to see that they were not entirely real. For example, he became fairly convinced that one of the other patient's visitors was stealing something and that was why they were leaving the building. Larry wanted to follow them until the police arrived. I was able to facilitate him to understand that this was not happening. I did this by using questions that required him to work out the logic of what was happening. At no time did I tell him that he was imaging things. I assumed that Larry was not so disturbed to have lost his problem-solving skills. This led Larry to identify that he was having 'dreams' thus demonstrating he had insight into his situation.

I wrote this up as an SI. The interaction strategies were very important and needed to be communicated to other nurses so they could build on my work, rather than having to work out such dynamics for themselves each time they came on duty. This type of intervention could not be prescribed as it involved reflection-in-action as I intuitively went along. The SI stated:

> *Larry is experiencing some 'dreams' which are causing him to feel distressed. During his dreams Larry is fully awake. How can we best work with Larry to help him through these dreams? Please make a note of any interventions or strategies that seem to help him.*

I then documented the interventions I had found useful. I expected the primary nurse to review the interventions, perhaps discuss with me and amend it as appropriate. All nurses in fact who worked with Larry added helpful interventions as well as evaluating previous written ones, thus testing them further in practice and evaluating them.

THE STRESS OF USING THE BURFORD MODEL

I identified four potential areas of stress from my perspective of being a full-time associate nurse. I feel that it is important to highlight these to create a balance as the previous ideas have been so positive.

1. Involvement

   The involvement demanded from the practitioner in their relationship with the patient/family. To be a holistic practitioner involves mutual sharing and the emotional energy stemming from this can be very draining for the practitioner. I assume that a nurse has only a finite amount of energy, and this is consumed at work, then home life may suffer and vice versa.

For example: Fred was admitted to Burford following a cerebral infarct which left him blind and confused. His wife, Agnes, was distraught – they had always been dependent on each other, having had no children and she was exhibiting signs that she could not see a future without Fred. For this reason she only left the hospital to sleep and expected intensive input from nursing staff all day and night which was not always possible to give with other patients' demands.

Agnes's stress levels meant that she had unrealistic expectations of the input we could give, both physically and emotionally. She would interrupt lunch breaks, telephone calls, work with other patients, and even impinge on off-duty time, for example, stopping my car as I left the car park to go home and telephoning staff at home. Reflecting on how this affected myself and listening to other staff talking it was obvious that Agnes demanded so much of our energy at work that home life was suffering: partners were becoming irritable because they did not want to hear again about Agnes and Fred. Social life was suffering as few of us had the inclination to do much except sleep once we had left work. Consequently our working practice began to suffer as resentment to Agnes became apparent. My energy reserves were drained with resultant feelings of guilt realising that I was not working in tune with our holistic vision that I firmly believed in.

2. Primary nursing

Although this area of stress is easily resolved due to team dynamics, I feel it is appropriate to highlight it. If I, in my associate nurse role admit a patient in the absence of the primary nurse and begin to build a therapeutic relationship, do I relinquish this on the return of the primary nurse? If so, I may feel cheated and undervalued and, if I do not, the primary nurse is placed in a dilemma of role definition. As I stated, this is usually overcome due to good peer working relationships. If I feel strongly about the relationship I have established with the patient, the primary nurse will often enable me to be that patient's primary nurse with support.

3. Access to one's own feelings

The reflective nature of the BNDU model encourages accessing one's own feelings, and although this is usually a positive stressor, at times it can be negative since awareness of feelings leads to actions upon them which may create further stress as the actions may not be easy to carry out. For example, I wrote

> *When the behaviour of a respite care patient changed such that it was causing stress for the daughter, her main carer, I realized that I resented the patient for upsetting the daughter. However, I did not wish to intervene and chose the easy option of observing the patient in order to 'pick up clues'. Through reflection and supervision I realized that this was not the most therapeutic response and was challenged as to whether I could or should confront the patient – not an easy action for me as I didn't wish to upset her.*[8]

4. Time

The BNDU model provides so much scope for good practice, but it does not provide any more hours in the day! Consequently, work can be 'taken home' and may interfere with home life. Although as an associate nurse I may not bring home 'practical' work as the primary nurses sometimes do, I still have 'emotional fall-out' and 'problem-solving' work to do.

COPING WITH STRESS

Burford's vision of practice articulates the essential significance of the therapeutic team to reciprocate and sustain practitioners in holistic practice and to give and receive necessary mutual support. Hence, a key aspect of work is to both utilise and contribute to this work. Clearly where work creates stress then systems are needed to deal with it at work. It is not satisfactory to expect to take it home to deal with as best I can. Yet, experience has proved that it is not always achieved as personal concerns do sometimes get in the way, and I/we become resentful, angry and defensive with our colleagues. We are all too human sometimes.[9]

CREATIVITY

As we have illustrated, working within the framework of the BNDU model enabled us to become more creative in our practice. We feel this has immense benefits for both the patient and the nurse. For patients, their care becomes more personal, more individualised. Nurses become more focused on developing therapeutic relationships rather than doing things to patients (Alfano 1971). We believe that in the long term, more positive health outcomes are achieved by nurses through communicating effectively with patients than by getting through the jobs that need to be done. This is not to say that basic aspects of care are neglected. It is important that patients' needs for physical care are also met.[10]

It is not easy to be creative as we have been socialised into acceptance of rules and regulations, of policies and procedures that are not easy to 'break free' from as they have been embodied and reinforced in everyday practice (Melia 1987).[11] Traditional nursing education socialises nurses into acceptance – acceptance of rules and regulations, of policies and procedures. It is often problematic for nurses to break free from these constraints and move towards therapeutic person-centred care which requires nurses to think critically for themselves.

This is especially so for lone nurses trying to change their practice within a team of nurses who continue to practice in traditional nurse-centred ways. Creativity must be acknowledged and accepted by a team of nurses for creativity and holistic practice to be effective. Nurses need to trust each other and not become stressed because they are not all doing it the same way.[12]

Becoming creative is clearly a learning process that incorporates an understanding of different types of knowledge. Becoming sensitive to problems, recognising disharmonies and making guesses suggests that knowledge other than research-based scientific knowledge is of value. This understanding validates the usefulness of constructed knowledge (Belenkey et al. 1986)[13] and sources of knowledge described as aesthetic and personal (Carper 1978).[14] Aesthetic knowledge is the 'art of nursing' (Vaughan 1992) that involves the assimilation of multiple sources of knowledge, notably intuition, in response to a particular situation. Personal knowing includes developing self-awareness and self-understanding. We have found that reflection facilitates our development of self-knowing. This is one of the reasons we emphasise the use of reflection and reflective techniques within the BNDU model in supporting our development and practice with our patients.

NOTES

1 I explore primary nursing roles in chapter 5 – a system for organising delivery of care.

2 You would imagine Kate would simply juxtapose her knowledge of Roper, Logan and Tierney Activities of living model alongside the cue – 'How has this event affected this person's normal life patterns and roles?' here 'life patterns' is akin to 'activities of living' yet without spelling them out. Kate's difficulty suggests how models frame reality and, as such, not so easily juxtaposed as I suggest. If nurse training focused on holistic care then it would make sense to teach the BNDU model (alongside other models) so that a cultural shift would be more evident. Nurses would then naturally be reflective and thoughtful, able to see the bigger picture rather than the limited picture framed by activities of living.

3 Kate notes how Transactional Analysis helped her cope with her feelings of being humiliated and in doing so accepting a 'child role' when appropriate. I have described this as 'tuning into the other's wavelength and flowing with it' rather than trying to force the person into your own wavelength which may not be therapeutic. It requires both understanding and humility to accept the 'child' role. Imagine most people's riposte – 'how dare he treat me like a child!'.

I first described this in 2004 in the second edition of becoming a reflective practitioner. The idea was inspired by Newman (1999) who described this tuning as 'synchronicity, a rhythm of relating in a paradigm of wholeness' I noted it was the caring dance, where each step a caring movement sometimes led by the practitioner and at other times by the other as appropriate (Johns 2001). Appreciating wavelength theory is an essential aspect of holistic practice.

I refer the reader back to page.

4 Jan's comment reflects how assessment is intended to be a continuous process of appreciating, reflecting and evaluating the person's shifting journey through their health-illness experience. In other words, it is not a one-off as often interpreted by non-holistic models.

5 Jan highlights the perverse and pervasive habit of labeling a person in negative terms – so that becomes the dominant lens to view the person with expectation that the patient will behave in that way. See literature...

6 I would add to Jan's list the way using a Special Intervention sheet highlights attention to specific aspects of care. Sometimes issues can get lost within the Reflexive narrative or passed over as not particularly significant.

7 This case study illustrates the creative response to the cue – 'How can I help this person?' It challenges the practitioner to see beyond their normal horizons to see the whole person and therapeutic options that may be beyond the practitioner's current skill mix. On reflection, the practitioner is challenged to consider other ways of responding using the Model for Structured Reflection cue – given the situation again could I respond more effectively in tune with my holistic vision? The guide (for example Jan) might say – 'have you considered aromatherapy?' The practitioner may say 'No... but tell me more' opening up the possibility to gain such skill of deemed appropriate. As it was Jan had such skill and could teach the practitioner.

8 Kate's sharing this in guided reflection over a series of sessions is shown on pages to illustrate guided reflection.

9 Kate and Jan note that the BNDU model pays explicit attention to the therapeutic team whereby practitioners are available to support one another and deal openly with conflict – this is addressed in the internal environment of care (see Chapter 1). Being available to colleagues reciprocates Being available to the person receiving care. Note that two attributes of 'Being available' are 'concern' and 'poise'. Hence a major focus of practitioner development is to nurture concern and strengthen poise – a fine balance whereas the 'therapeutic team' is the environment where being available becomes possible reinforced by reflection and supervision.

10 The BNDU model views the whole person and their whole needs. There is no priority given to any aspect of care. The idea of 'basic' aspects of care is spurious. It is a relic or hangover from previous ways of practice.

11 Hence the vital need to create a supportive culture where these constraints can be understood and shed like an old skin and where nurses can think and reflect critically about realising the BNDU vision as a lived reality with appropriate support through guidance. It is the key role of the leader with foresight to facilitate this.

12 Hence, the necessity for a collective vision is vital to give direction and purpose to practice and as a reminder to practitioners if and when they do not pull together. As such, creating a valid vision is the first step to becoming creative and holistic.

13 Belenkey et al. developed a typology of voice that offers a practical framework for practitioners development of voice towards communicative competence (as I set out in Chapter 4).

14 I used the work of Carper to initially frame insights gained through learning through reflection. I replaced this with the Being Available template. See Johns C (2022) becoming 'reflective practitioner (sixth edition) Wiley Blackwell, Oxford (Chapter 5 - pages 52–58).

REFERENCES

Alfano G (1971) Healing or caretaking - which will it be. *Clinics of North America* 6(2); 273–80.

Belenkey M F, Clinchy B M, Goldberger N R, and Tarule J M (1986) *Women's ways of knowing*. Basic Books, New York.

Berne E (1964) *Games people play; the psychology of human relationships*. Penguin, London.

Carper B (1978) Fundamental ways of knowing in nursing. *Advances in Nursing Science* 1(1); 13–23.

Johns C (1991) The Burford Nursing Development Unit holistic model of nursing practice. *Journal of Advanced Nursing* 16; 1090–98.

Johns C (2001) The caring dance. *Complementary Therapies in Nursing and Midwifery* 7(1); 8–12.

Manthey M (1980) *The practice of primary nursing*. Blackwell Scientific Publications, Oxford.

Melia K (1987) *Learning and working – the occupational socialization of nursing*. Tavistock Publications, London.

Newman M (1999) The rhythm of relating in a paradigm of wholeness. *Image: Journal of Nursing Scholarship* 31; 227–30.

Pearson A (1988) *Primary nursing: nursing in the Oxford and Burford nursing development units*. Chapman Hall, London.

Salvage J (1990) Introduction. In *Models for Nursing, 2* (Eds. J Salvage and B Kershaw) Scutari Press, Harrow.

Vaughan B (1992) The nature of nursing knowledge. In *Knowledge for nursing practice* (Eds. K Robinson and B Vaughan) Butterworth Heinemann, Oxford.

The BNDU Model in Use at the Oxford Community Hospital

CHAPTER 11

Brendan McCormack, Carol McCaffrey and Susan Booker

This chapter has three main intentions:

1. To utilise the supporting themes of the BNDU model in order to describe the context in which the model was used in a specific practice environment
2. To highlight a particular case to describe the utility of the model in practice
3. Using a particular theoretical framework, to offer a critical analysis of the appropriateness of the model for practice

THE SETTING IN CONTEXT

The four key components of the philosophy for practice as described by Johns (1991) and from which the BNDU holistic model was developed are:

- External environment of care
- Internal environment of care
- Social viability
- The nature of care

ENVIRONMENT OF CARE

The emphasis of the BNDU holistic model is practice and because practice is rooted in an environment which is both unstable and unpredictable, then the need to 'capture the reality of practice and the beliefs and values of the practitioners' is paramount. This tension between the espoused ideology and the ideology as lived in practice, and its resultant effect on patient

Holistic Practice in Healthcare: The Burford NDU Person-centred Model, Second Edition. Edited by Christopher Johns.

care has been recently documented by Ahmed and Kitson (1992). These authors concluded that the tension between the two ideologies led to inconsistent and discontinuous care patterns. It is not new for nurse theorists to address environmental issues in their development of nursing models, (for example Roper et al. 1980, Roy 1989, Orem 1980). Indeed, Roper et al. (1980:30) state

> *Environmental factors cannot be considered in isolation; they are related to physical, psychological and socio-cultural... and also to politico-economic factors...*

However, in addressing environmental issues, Roper et al. discuss such topics as the atmosphere, sunrays, light rays, sound waves, and atmospheric components. While these are certainly important factors in our everyday living and our health status, they are not the issues that immediately come to mind in everyday practice (Benner and Wrubel 1989, Melia 1990). The BNDU model attempts to address more local environmental issues. These will now be discussed in the authors' area of practice.

EXTERNAL ENVIRONMENT OF CARE

The external environment relates to the context and function of the particular nursing practice (Johns 1991) and the philosophy must be relevant to the context of where care is carried out (Johns 1990).

Oxford Community hospital (OXCOMM) is not an independent building, but situated within the structure of a large general hospital. It serves a predominantly elderly population (although not designated and elderly care area) in a local environment with a range of services from rehabilitation, respite care for the chronically sick, care of the dying and day hospital assessment and treatment. These services are centred around an operational philosophy which states:

> *... Oxford Community hospital should function as an integral part of the community health services with an emphasis on the maintenance and resettlement of people in their 'home' environment*

This approach to service delivery is consistent with Tucker's (1987) comment that 'the Community hospital serves the community and is served by the community'. Indeed, the NHS Health Advisory Service (NHS 1991) recognises that the community hospitals of Oxfordshire are ideally placed to be developed as 'multi-disciplinary, multi-agency resource centres with full access for local residents, sub-serving the social, physical and mental health needs of elderly people'.[1] The hospital is actively involved in developing an outreach philosophy and the strengthening of links between primary and secondary care.

INTERNAL ENVIRONMENT OF CARE

The internal environment is concerned with issues such as relationships between nurses and with other health professionals (Johns 1991).

The organisation of nursing at OXCOMM is based on the philosophy of primary nursing. Each patient admitted is allocated a named nurse, known as a primary nurse, who is responsible for the coordination of care for that patient within the multi-disciplinary team. This organisational philosophy has been in practice since the inception of the unit and is an established ideology amongst practitioners. However, issues relating to role ambiguity and confusion are evident in the hospital and, due to the number of staff employed and the irregular hours worked, practical difficulties in maintaining open and honest lines of communication exist. Behaviour which characterises this culture includes (McCormack 1993)

- Giving and receiving feedback
- Maintaining interpersonal diplomacy
- Withholding feelings
- Suppressing anger
- Hurt, suspicion and mistrust

We postulate that a model of 'living' must offer a way of describing what 'living' means. Whilst recognising that most people would describe everyday activities such as eating, drinking and sleeping as essential to life, many philosophical issues of living may also be seen as important. Indeed Watson (1985) argues that

> *a humanistic-altruistic value system is a qualitative philosophy that guides one's life.*

And it is this value system that:

> *... helps one tolerate differences and to view others through their own perceptual systems rather than through one's own.*

It is difficult to capture this individual phenomenological approach to experience within a model that focuses on body systems. The model of living does not easily transfer assessment of needs to an individualised holistic plan of care.

Roper et al.'s model conforms to a linear model of analysis. However, more contemporary work suggests that decision-making in nursing does not necessarily adhere to the linear model but instead incorporates a more intuitive, holistic mode of thinking (Pyles and Stern 1983, Benner 1984, Young 1987). Furthermore, adherence to a formal linear model of practice devalues intuitive knowledge as a legitimate component of scientific method and fails to recognise holistic modes of thinking (McCormack 1992). The work of Benner (1984) has initiated the redressing of the emphasis on linear models of thinking and problem-solving, thereby causing a shift towards more holistic modes.

THE NATURE OF CARE

The nature of care is primarily concerned with the relationship between the nurse and the patient. Within the influences and constraints of the environment (Johns 1991).

Nurses at OXCOMM place value on the individuality of the person receiving care while recognising the problematic nature of *working with* patients. Issues relating to the complexities of preserving and understanding patient autonomy and patients' rights to choice, raise practical and emotional concerns for nurses. Smith (1992) in her research with student nurses concluded that emotional components of care require formal and systematic training to manage feelings.

Egan (1990) argues that helpers who do not understand themselves can inflict a great deal of harm on their clients. Therefore, the importance of nurses being 'self-aware' is paramount in an organisation that centres its practice on the therapeutic nurse-patient relationship.

Nurses need to be aware of their motives for caring. Clearly there are professional motives involved, as a basic tenet of being professional is the ability to be self-regulating, i.e. reflecting on practice and re-evaluating outcomes. Through this process practitioners can identify deficiencies in their practice and organise approaches for change. The BNDU model offers the client an opportunity to be involved in the self-regulating process, as its structure and focus promotes active involvement of the patient in their care management.

It can be concluded therefore that the BNDU holistic model is appropriate for this particular practice setting. While we are currently developing an explicitly stated set of values and beliefs in the form of a philosophy for practice, the principles which nursing staff articulate in their practice are compatible with this expressed in the BNDU model. The articulation of these beliefs and values is recognised as a continuous process in the development of patient-centred practice in this unit.

THE MODEL IN USE: CASE STUDY OF EVA

The BNDU model is not yet widely used at OXCOMM but one that practitioners are becoming more familiar with. In this case study the implementation of the BNDU model in practice was a joint decision between the patient and her carers. The authors were functioning as joint care-givers to the patient (Eva). The relationship between the authors was of student (Carol), mentor (Sue) and teacher (Brendan). Pyles and Stern (1983) recognise that the mentor (an experienced nurse) has a key function to play in the socialisation of student nurses. The mentor acts as a teacher, advisor, counsellor and role model for the novice nurse.

The role of the teacher is that of helping the students to identify, explore and expand on their own latent knowledge (Miller and Rew 1989) in the practice setting. The teacher facilitates the students to develop and reflect on their intuitive and objective knowledge. It is essential that the teacher is seen to 'struggle' to solve problems with the student rather than only providing answers. While recognising the use of problem-solving through linear analysis, the learner needs to be able to look deeper at problems and recognise that not all cases and problems can fit into mechanistic frameworks. Therefore problem-solving strategies that focus on the question rather than the answer were employed in this case.

This approach gives further credibility to the value of feelings and beliefs in the nurse-patient relationship, thus counteracting Visintainer's (1986) view that nurses place little credibility on their feelings and beliefs –the 'soft stuff of nursing'. The work of Schon (1983) has begun the re-addressing of the essence of nursing through the reflective process. Indeed, the assessment strategy utilised in the BNDU model can be seen to be a model of reflection in itself with the starting point the cue –'What information do I need to nurse this person?'

In order to capture the essence of the relationship, sections from carol's reflective diary are included where appropriate. This approach further legitimises the use of the cue questions –'How does this person make me feel?' and 'How can I help this person?', by demonstrating the nature of the interactions that occurred in this nurse-patient relationship and their articulation through reflection.

ASSESSMENT OF EVA'S NEED FOR CARE

When Eva was admitted the decision not to read her medical notes was a conscious one, since it was preferred to let her present herself to her nurse, hence guarding against any expectations or preconceived ideas about her personality and her condition.

Assessment of Eva's needs was performed initially using Roper et al.'s model for nursing. While much valuable information was obtained, the process of acquiring this felt uncomfortable and intrusive for both Eva and Carol.

REFLECTION

The model is in my opinion very functional having used it to assess my patient. She is fortunately very open, talkative person who enjoys talking about her problems and how she sees the future for herself and her family. In order to get around the questions in Roper et al.'s model, I needed to use open questions and encourage her husband to participate in the assessment. The most difficult part was the assessment of sexuality. This was challenging for me, if not a little embarrassing. But Eva reassured me – 'Don't worry, I don't mind' – making me feel a little more at ease. Discussing death also proved unnerving. There was something not right about this experience.

A re-assessment of Eva's needs was performed using the BNDU model.

Instead of attempting to make underlying assumptions, the BNDU model allowed me to see Eva more in the context of her social and cultural world.

The Burford model assessment consists of one core question and a series of cues to tune the nurse into the philosophic concepts of the model (as opposed to the functional concepts). These cues have not been altered in any way from their original format as described by Johns (1991). While Johns' asserts that the cues do not require specific information, the assessment process in this study is presented in this way to demonstrate the utility of the model.

WHO IS THIS PERSON?

Eva was the youngest and sole survivor of a family of four children and she had three children of her own; two daughters and one son, who all lived nearby and visited regularly. She had been married to John for 38 years and prior to her hospitalisation lived with him in purpose-built accommodation in Oxfordshire. A 69-year-old lady, she led an independent life until her disabilities overcame her physical ability to mobilise her independently.

WHAT HEALTH EVENT HAS BROUGHT THIS PERSON INTO HOSPITAL?

The aim of Eva's stay at OXCOMM was to help her after surgery of an abscess in her left lumbar region and to come to terms with the increasing severity of her debilitating rheumatoid arthritis. Her cavity wound was a result of taking steroid-based medication for this thirty-year-long illness. Eva was wheelchair-bound and is a diabetic. She was fighting to regain control of her consciousness, with increasing success following the removal of an indwelling catheter after almost four years in-situ.

HOW MUST THIS PERSON BE FEELING?

Eva once expressed to Carol that she felt that 'life is just one misery'. She was depressed at times, frightened that her wound would not heal quickly and exhausted by the fatigue of her arthritis caused her and the 'energy drained' feeling that she complained of, probably due to the medication that she was taking. She not only feared for her own future but also for John (her husband), who was very concerned about her and lonely at home without her.

HOW HAS THIS EVENT AFFECTED THIS PERSON'S NORMAL LIFE-PATTERN AND ROLES?

Eva's admission to OXCOMM affected her usual life pattern and roles minimally, since Eva's active roles had been very limited due to her crippling arthritis. She missed and yearned for the comfort and familiarity of her own home, John taking her for walks and tending to her plants. Eva's residual roles in her family were very strong. She was a very communicable person who said she was always 'ready for a chat'. She enjoyed airing her feelings, reminiscing about the past and reflecting often on the present and the uncertainty which the future held.

HOW DOES THIS PERSON MAKE ME FEEL?

On the whole, Eva made us feel good, the role as her nurse was highly rewarding and satisfying. Eva, despite being very physically dependent, was independent in spirit and willing to participate as much as she could in all aspects of her care. Her cooperation rarely faltered except on those days when her pain and fatigue overcame her. On such occasions Eva became passive and often self-pitying, at which time we felt great empathy towards her and a determination to cheer her up to make her stay as comfortable as possible.

HOW CAN I HELP THIS PERSON?

Eva was helped by planning the most effective health care based on our assessment of her capabilities and dependency. The care Eva needed was both clinical (in respect of her wound) and psychological, which involved interacting with her for long periods of time and giving her continuous encouragement and reassurance.[2]

WHAT IS IMPORTANT TO MAKE THIS PERSON'S STAY IN HOSPITAL COMFORTABLE?

1. Management of her pain. Eva described it as a 'round the clock' problem. Her pain was multi-focal and ranged on a Raiman scale from moderate to severe. Eva often complained of pains in her back, neck and had frequent headaches.

2. Care of her wound. Eva's wound caused her much distress resulting in her always asking 'how is it getting on?', when it was being redressed. She saw her wound as the main obstacle preventing her from returning home; hence, it was essential that we established an honest and open relationship, to allow her to come to terms with the severity of her illness, using a sensitive, positive approach.
3. Management of her continence and bowels. Although these may not to a diagnosing clinician stand out as either of Eva's main problems, they were her main concerns, causing her much anxiety. She was prone to constipation since she did not move around very much, and as a result she felt so 'bloated'. Having recently had a four-year catheter removed, Eva was concerned about maintaining her self-esteem, and was successfully regaining control of her continence.

WHAT SUPPORT DOES THIS PERSON HAVE?

Eva's primary support was her husband John. He proudly said 'I do everything for her when at home'. He did the washing, shopping and cooking, helping her up in the mornings and to bed at night. Although John felt very capable and said he was 'very fit', he suffered from angina and was often breathless upon coming to visit Eva. Nevertheless, he was very keen to get her back home, insisting that he could look after her with the assistance of a home help during the week and a girl from 'Crossroads', a home-care organisation, at weekends. But after much talking about the practicalities of dealing with Eva's wound care and pain, John mentioned his desire to get her home less often as did Eva herself.

HOW DO THEY VIEW THE FUTURE FOR THEMSELVES AND OTHERS?

Eva described her current illness as 'the last straw' and often expressed that 'I just don't know what's going to happen next.' Since her operation to have her wound sutured, and with much counselling Eva had come to realise that she and John could not cope alone at home. She certainly wished to return home and to regain some of her independence which would require a lot of willpower and motivation not only on her part but that of her husband. She said 'I don't know what I would do without John' giving us the impression that if he was gone she would give up the will to live.

PLANNING AND GIVING CARE

Due to the patient-centred approach of the assessment process, it seemed appropriate to use metaphors to describe the planning and implementation of care. Following assessment of Eva's needs, a 'priorities of care' list was drawn up with Eva (Figure 11.1) using Neuman's levels of nursing interventions as proposed in the BNDU model (Johns 1991).[3]

Problem: 'I've had my fill of hospitals'
Focus of problem: loss of self-esteem and depression

Eva openly expressed her negative feelings about being at the community hospital. She said she was sick of being in hospital and would prefer to be cared for at home where she could do 'her own thing'. And be with John. In our recognition that this was impossible at present, we did realise that it was especially important for Eva's wound to heal quickly, and by giving her lots of support throughout her stay we aimed to allow her to return home as soon as possible.

Eva's admission undoubtedly had psychological and social implications for her; her removal from her home environment and her missing husband were contributing factors.

Primary interventions

1. Preparation of Eva to return to her own home with John as her main carer.
2. Preparation of John for Eva's discharge home and equipping him with the necessary skills to care for her
3. Promotion of Eva's self-esteem by reinforcing a positive self-image while caring for her

Secondary interventions

1. Wound care
2. Control of Eva's diabetes and promotion of wound healing through the provision of adequate nutrition
3. Control of Eva's pain including massage

Tertiary interventions

1. Control of Eva's incontinence
2. Support for John in his caring role

FIGURE 11.1 Priorities of care based on Neuman's typology (1980)

REFLECTION

I understand the concept of the patient's experience as a crucial element of the philosophy of care. It is necessary to focus on and understand what the illness event means to Eva and her family; hence the importance of taking her assessment and viewing her as a member of the community with a social and cultural world, and centring nursing action around her needs from a holistic perspective that recognises the uniqueness of her personal experience.

One evening upon entering her room, we heard her say to her husband 'I just look so awful.' He reassured her that this was not the case, but she remained unconvinced. It could be suggested therefore that she was grieving for the loss of body image, a consequence of her deteriorating arthritis and her ever-increasing problems with mobility, resulting in her low self-esteem and lack of social roles. Either way, we recognised that time, patience and understanding were of the essence when delivering care to Eva. Having implemented this in the care plan, we felt that perhaps the carers could accept her depression as a 'natural process' of expressing her grief.

Problem: 'my back is killing me'
Focus of problem: wound care and maintenance of Eva's autonomy

The dimensions of the wound and its location contributed to Eva's discomfort especially on physical exertion, and indeed, she reiterated this on a number of occasions. 'My back is killing me' she would often say, accounting not only for her physical discomfort but also for her depression for which she took daily medication.

The need for Eva's wound was to heal quickly required selection of a suitable dressing since inappropriate selection can often increase pain (Thomas 1989). A thorough assessment of the wound was completed. A calcium-alginate-based ribbon dressing to pack her wound daily was used, with the knowledge that the predicted rapid and pain-free healing process employed would help Eva make a speedy recovery which would assist in improving her social roles.

Care of Eva's wound involved irrigation, assessment and redressing daily. We allowed Eva to decide the time when this procedure was performed. In doing this we felt that we were not disturbing her usual routine which was important as she felt anxious and depressed at times, and appreciation of her wanting to have a 'lie-in' could warrant her feeling more at home and at ease during her stay. This approach was appropriate for her and Eva was able to plan her day in advance with John.

REFLECTION

I was reminded of this quote from Forster (1989) which reflected the complexity of preserving patient autonomy:

When my time comes I'm not going to allow it
When my time comes I won't trust to mystery
When my time comes I will say I have had enough and go
That is, if my time comes like Granma's time
If it is the same sort of time
But if it is, I won't be able to, will I?
Problem: 'Do I have to eat all this?'

Focus of problem: control of Eva's diabetes and promotion of wound healing through the provision of an appropriate diet

Congruent with Eva's wound management was the need for her to be well nourished. She was a diet-controlled diabetic and had been for 'a couple of years now'. In the knowledge that diabetes is the most common condition that may account for delayed wound healing due to defective carbohydrate and fat metabolism (Ross and Benditt 1962), Eva's 'BM stix' was recorded twice daily. Ross and Benditt's study emphasised the need for normal protein metabolism.

Following a long chat with Eva, we all agreed that she should commence a high protein diet. Eva had complained on several occasions about her food. 'It's awful' she said. This helped her accept a special diet, and she was pleased to have special soups and yoghurts sent from the kitchen in addition to the sugar-free extras (drinks, fruit and sweets) brought by John nearly every evening. When asked how she was eating she replied 'Very well. The food seems to have improved.'

We did not feel the need to reinforce Eva's nutrition patterns however. Following discussion with her, we emphasised the importance of continuing this regime on her return home, knowing that the slightest possibility of readmission would upset Eva and John a great deal.

Both were adamant that they would stick to the present regime, John reassuring us that he would 'keep an eye on her'.

REFLECTION

This approach to Eva's care reinforces the importance of partnership in the nurse-patient relationship. Through focusing on the cue question – 'who is this person?', it remained paramount to always allow Eva to take the lead in organizing her care delivery.[4]

Problem: 'I feel so bruised and tender that life is just one misery'

Focus of problem: control of Eva's pain

Parallel to and precipitated by Eva's wound care was her multi-focal pain. Eva found any form of movement difficult and painful especially her neck that felt bruised and tender. It was obvious that she was in pain upon mobilising, not only via her verbal cues but also her agonised facial expression and the gasps which seemed to take the breath from her. From Eva's perspective, it was felt that by allowing her to monitor her pain and giving her some autonomy, she would think more objectively about it, thus allowing an opportunity for us all to set the most appropriate goals for the future. More importantly, the mere fact that Eva could see that we were taking her pain seriously could perhaps make her feel better.

REFLECTION

On a few occasions I have found myself in the situation where an elderly patient has complained of pain and I have thought 'she's looking for attention' or 'it can't be that bad!' later I felt ashamed of myself for delaying the patient their autonomy and individuality, whilst denying myself the opportunity to fulfil my role as a partner in what should be a 'mutual trust' relationship with my patient.[5]

Eva's previous experience of pain and the anxiety that she experienced regarding admission to hospital were clearly associated with pain ratings. On those days when Eva expressed feeling down or depressed, she complained of more pain. Indeed, Bond (1984) states that such anxiety can often intensify pain.

One particular day when Eva expressed that 'life is just one misery' her pain ratings were higher than usual and she described her pain as 'unbearable'. Hence we felt the need to spend talking with Eva, giving her information regarding her pain and its control. The mutual trust relationship we had established enabled more effective recognition of anxiety-evoking stimuli that were affecting her. We felt we were making contact with Eva's feelings and concerns, thereby learning from her and developing our clinical knowledge (knowing).[6]

This example clearly illustrates the concept of 'situated meaning' whereby the patient does not respond to the situation solely in terms of what they have lost, but instead continues to be engaged by concerns, meanings and even a limited future (Benner and Wrubel 1989).

Eva spoke of 'missing John' of 'feeling so useless', concerned about the present and future likelihood of her recovery to full health. 'I just don't know what's going to happen to me' she once said. By allowing John open visiting hours, and using Eva's own bed linen as well as the homely comforts of radio and TV in her room, we felt we could make Eva more comfortable in her present surroundings and less concerned about the future.

Eva always preferred to leave her bedroom door open so she could see 'what was going on', hence often attracting the attention of a passer-by, to whom she would complain of pain followed by sleepless nights. Whether or not these were due to a noisy environment (besides the nurses' station) or her temazepan-controlled insomnia, we were not sure. Mullooly (1988) has suggested that patients report less pain when nurses in quiet surroundings. Eva had 'settled in well now' and we felt it would be unfair to move her to another room. We did feel though that this could be taken into consideration upon any future admissions to the unit, although (when given the choice) Eva said she preferred the room she was in.

We found that distracting activities seemed to be effective in controlling Eva's pain. She would sit for long periods doing a puzzle or watching TV and never talked about pain or discomfort. However, the family influence was significant. When John visited her pain behaviour increased and we often had to help him to turn her in bed. The literature suggests this was not uncommon (Hosking and Welchew 1985); hence, we accepted this as one of Eva's characteristics. However, not all staff were able to see it this way and this sometimes resulted in their demonstration of controlling behaviour towards Eva.

REFLECTION

I found it interesting to note my feelings of protection and advocacy when this was being discussed negatively by other staff. Confronting them about their attitude was easier said than done and I often tended to just say nothing in the hope that their conversation would soon end.[7]

In order to reduce Eva's pain during the redressing of her wound that was 'so painful', we decided a massage session might be of benefit. She expressed willingness to have her lower legs massaged using aromatherapy oils. We talked through the procedure, encouraging her to concentrate on the massage. The outcome was rewarding and Eva spoke of how much she enjoyed the session.

REFLECTION

By initiating these massage sessions, I felt as if I had developed my communication skills with her, not just verbally but now non-verbally. The outcome for me was more than rewarding – she spoke on several occasions of how much she enjoyed the sessions. I feel an outcome for both of us was a feeling of being 'cared for'. For her, the benefits were two-fold; the release of her emotions and buried feelings as her tensed muscles and aching joints were soothed, providing obvious contentment and feelings of well-being. Secondly, the attention was detracted from the wound as was mine and Eva's aim. I received feedback from other nurses that Eva asked after me and said how kind I was and how much she enjoyed my massage sessions. Making the decisions about her present and future were made easier by this relationship.

There was little doubt that Eva's pain would be ever present on her return home and it was necessary to encourage her to keep occupied as much as possible. John was very protective over her and tended to do everything for her. She missed doing the chores and went on to say 'now John has to do them all'. We encouraged a more participative role in her lifestyle as this could increase Eva's morale and feeling of having the pain under control enabling her to play a more active role both physically and socially.

Eva said she felt 'so useless now'. Her interests were all passive, she enjoyed reading, watching TV and doing puzzles. She said she used to make a cake every time her son came around to see her but was 'not able to do so now'. We found ourselves questioning her abilities. Was she physically unable or was she simply not given the initiative to take more active roles? Discussion with Eva reassured us that we could eliminate her pain as the cause of her lack of inactivity.

REFLECTION

> *This I must appreciate and understand, since the threat of any potential pain would obviously prove too much, and, further, she is uncertain as to what the future holds for her; she is unsure about when she will return home, if ever she reaches a recovery state as acceptable to her, where pain and immobility are nor prevalent.*

Problem: 'Paving the way to self-control'

Focus of problem: control of continence

Eva's concerns with her bowels and her continence were hardly surprising since she recently had a four-year indwelling catheter removed. She also suffered from constipation as a result of poor muscle tone and limited mobility and possibly as one of the side effects of her medication. Eva had become very upset on a few occasions about how she 'cannot go herself', but was willing to have an enema every two days to relieve her discomfort. Having re-established a routine, she began to go on her own, and she felt this was great.

By establishing a continence programme for Eva she was going less often. Initially, after removal of the catheter Eva was using her commode almost every hour passing large amounts of urine. Later, she regained control of her micturition and often did not ask for a commode for at least two hours at a time. We spent a lot of time educating and reassuring Eva especially when helping her to get up in the mornings, explaining that her lack of control was to be expected, but she always just said 'I wish I could go on my own, like everybody else.'

EVALUATION OF CARE AND ACHIEVING OUTCOMES

From a physical perspective Eva presented us with a plethora of needs that complicated each other. However, we reached a mutually satisfying conclusion. Our aim whilst working with her as to recognise her real potential within the hospital's rehabilitation philosophy

> *We believe that OCCOMM should offer a rehabilitation service, based on the assumption that clients will ultimately be discharged to another setting whilst recognizing that this process may, for some people take a long time.*

Throughout her care programme, Eva's holistic care needs were met and no need was viewed in isolation. The BNDU model offered the opportunity to achieve this through its focus on philosophical concepts rather than the activities of living. However, the model does appear to lack any structural direction to the planning of care and evaluation of outcomes other than stating that the model *rejects any determinism that manifests itself by stating goals in terms of what the patient will achieve without patient involvement. (Johns 1991)*

The setting of goals in this model does take a patient-centred approach, so therefore one assumes that it is the patient's perspective that determines when goals have been achieved. This phenomenological approach to assessment and care planning is one that as yet would be unfamiliar to most nurses, and be one of the reasons why this model may be rejected by practitioners without appropriate support to facilitate the cultural and attitudinal change. Without this cultural paradigm shift practitioners may never achieve the full potential of the model by relying on (previous) linear approaches to problem identification rooted in a functional perspective.

Evaluation of the outcomes of Eva's care centred around a daily evaluation of care compared to Eva's long-term objectives. Eva's own comments were used as part of this evaluation process and agreement was reached when changes in the direction of care were required. This process facilitated the communication of Eva's social-psycho needs and minimised the regression towards evaluation of physical care centred on activities of living. If patient autonomy is to be really respected, then it would seem appropriate for nurses to legitimise the value of patients' comments, interactions, and discussions by utilising their actual words rather than our interpretations of them.[8]

CRITIQUE OF THE BNDU MODEL

The debate about the usefulness or not of nursing models is one that continues to preoccupy theoreticians and the nursing press. Indeed, in the pursuit of academia, nursing models have been used as the foundation for the development of theoretical principles. While the majority of these theoretical advancements fall into the conceptual model category (Kristjanson et al. 1987), their usefulness for guiding practice has been limited. Many of these models need further exploration of their espoused theoretical principles and their relationship and relevance to nursing practice.

Evaluation of theory is an essential component of nursing practice and of knowledge development (Meleis 1991) who offers a comprehensive framework for the evaluation of theory in nursing. This framework will be utilised to critique the BNDU model and identify development issues.

CLARITY

The BNDU holistic model of nursing practice clearly articulates its underlying concepts, values and beliefs. These have been developed from practice with a focus on the articulation of internal beliefs and values. This focus arose from the belief that the imposition of an external philosophy is conceptually problematic due to its potential conflict with practitioners' own beliefs and values.

The BNDU model poses a similar problem, as without the articulation of a practice area's beliefs and values the model is difficult to integrate in practice. The case study of Eva highlights that the model is suitable on an individual level when a similar ideology is espoused.

However, in order for its process to be accepted on a wider scale, cultural beliefs and values of the hospital would need to be explicitly stated in order to create a shift towards more patient-centred practice. The experience of using the BNDU model suggests that it can assist this process as it offers direction for development to the practitioner. As such, the BNDU model can encapsulate the collective beliefs and values of a group of practitioners, while freeing the individual practitioner from the shackles of conformity to a set of values that they may not espouse.

CONSISTENCY

Meleis (1991) describes consistency as the degree which congruence exists between the different components of a theory. The BNDU model would appear to be consistent in its approach and the core and cue questions (of its assessment strategy) offer clear direction or both assessment and organisation of care.

The humanistic and holistic concepts articulated in the model are reflected through the assessment process. However, lack of structure in goal setting could be problematic for the widespread adoption of this framework.

The concept of 'therapeutic interventions' would appear to require further exploration and clarification due to the weakness of the approach to evaluation. Johns (1991) asserts that the word 'therapeutic' refers to nursing actions for the benefit of the patient within a focus of patient-centred needs. Hockey (1991) argues that the way in which one views the possibilities of therapeutic nursing or what one identifies as the activity of therapeutic nursing clearly depends on one's interpretation of it. If this is the case, then the BNDU model offers an enormous challenge to nurses and nursing and places even greater importance on the explicit statement of beliefs and values in nursing.

Many of the principles explicated in the BNDU model are appropriate to inform OXCOMM practice due to similarities in the nature of the service and patient focus. The philosophical beliefs are compatible with those of OXCOMM practitioners. And to this end the BNDU model may act as a useful tool to guide the articulation of those beliefs and values in the form of a philosophy.[9]

SIMPLICITY

The underlying concepts of the BNDU model are relatively simple to understand and implement in practice. Chin and Jacobs (1987) argue for simplicity in theory, but caution against simplicity in untested theory.[10]

The model could be seen as deceptively simple in its construction as many of the underlying principles are complex and problematic to implement in practice due to internal and external organisational constraints. Principles such as 'holism', 'reciprocity', and 'working with' are concepts that are not yet understood by nurses and indeed, are often negated due to attitudinal and organisational constraints.

However, the BNDU model is easy to describe and uses language that is familiar to nurses. For this reason, the BNDU model has potential to act as a framework to aid the development of nursing practice and the articulation of therapeutic patient outcomes.

USEFULNESS

Some would suggest that the whole issues of nursing models has served a negative purpose in the advancement of nursing knowledge (Meleis 1991, Robinson 1990) and has detracted from the real issues in nursing, i.e. the theory-practice gap.

Meleis (1991) takes a more objective approach to the issues of nursing models and theory development and suggests that nursing is in a state of transition from that of practice, with its focus on routine and subservience, through the education and administration, and research stages, to the present position of theory, where the development of nursing knowledge rooted in practice is paramount. She suggests that contrary to other evolutionary or revolutionary developments, nursing progress seems to have charted its own path with previously rejected ideas being accepted at later stages.

A clear example of this lies within the BNDU model, whereby the concept of environment is central to the model's focus – a concept that was widely discussed by Nightingale and which was subsequently rejected by positive science. It is within this development of 'theory of practice' that this model is firmly rooted as applied in the case study of Eva.

Meleis (1991) suggests that a theory should be useful in all areas of nursing: practice, research, education and administration. The BNDU model has the potential to be useful in all these areas. Through the use of the BNDU model it has been possible to identify areas that need development in the practice setting. The importance of developing a philosophy for practice is one such area, as is the need to address organisational issues that negate against patient-centred practice. This is perhaps the greatest asset of the BNDU model.

CONCLUSIONS

The implementation of the BNDU model in practice has proven to be a challenge both conceptually and emotionally. We felt drawn closer to the patient through the assessment process and patient-centred approach to implementing the care programme.

While no deliberate attempt was made to alter the structure of the BNDU model for the purpose of this exercise, further work with the model through the articulation of a philosophy for practice will no doubt raise challenges to explore. This dynamic approach is refreshing as it enables the model to come 'alive' in the practice setting and grow and develop through patients' and practitioners' experiences. Indeed, as Meleis (1991:147) suggests

> *As we nurture our emerged identity, we need to support more coherent approaches to knowledge development; ones that encompass knowing, understanding and caring; ones that support the development of models of knowledge development congruent with our mission.*

NOTES

1 The very same statement could be made today regarding the crisis with social care and bed blocking in general hospitals.

2 To make the point that the BNDU model from its holistic perspective would view no distinction between 'clinical' and 'psychological' or

indeed any other category of being. I sense this is a hangover from the medical model whereby 'clinical' (focusing on physical aspects of care) is observed, valued and lends itself to the application of specific knowledge-based action in contrast with the more invisible aspects of care such as what might be deemed 'psychological' that tends to be complex and indeterminate and elusive to specific action.

3 See my comment on page – regarding my decision to discontinue using Neuman's schema.

4 The key to communication within the nurse-patient relationship is dialogue – whereby the perspectives and preconceptions of the practitioner are suspended to enable the patient to express their own expectations, fears and such like, leading to a mutual understanding of each other's thoughts and negotiation to agree the best a way forward which may not be the patient's most desired way – see chapter 4.

5 This reflection highlights the negative attitude that practitioners can have and which constrain holistic practice. It also highlights the power of reflection to confront self in light of one's beliefs about the nature of practice and to ask and investigate 'where the negative attitude stem from?' Perhaps we have to feel the same as a trigger and energy for change. The insight is profound and life changing revealing the necessity for guided reflection as an essential developmental process towards realising holistic practice. Having a vision is one thing, realising it is quite another – see pages....

6 I have bracketed the word 'knowing' in contrast with knowledge to make the distinction that reflection leads to development of practical knowing rather than knowledge which is something more abstract and can be applied. Knowing is what subconsciously guides one's perceptions and actions – see pages.

7 From a leadership perspective, this type of situation is common when first implementing the BNDU model – when beliefs and values may not be shared by all practitioners and 'old ways' of viewing people as objects remain prevalent. Hence the importance of the shared vision. As a leader I might encourage the practitioner to raise the issues of attitudes towards Eva at handover of care or raise it myself by asking 'how do we feel about Eva' mindful of the need for shifts of attitude and the practitioner's concern. The experience illustrates the existence of the harmonious team (see page) whereby feelings are not easily shared and situations of conflict hard to deal with and hence 'brushed under the carpet'. Creating the therapeutic team is fundamental to realising holistic practice.

8 Some points:

   1 Evaluation of care is a continuous narrative process through an on-going cycle of assessment, planning, action and evaluation. It is a dynamic form rather than the static linear flow of the nursing process.
   2 The 'problems' identified for Eva may be recorded on Special Intervention sheets (see page...) to highlight the 'problem' from the general narrative.
   3 The use of the patient's own words is very desirable from a narrative perspective because it 'lights-up' who the person is. The use of metaphors is a very creative approach and again 'lights-up' the humanity of the person and caring.
   4 The use of massage again illustrates the creativity of the nurse who is open to new ideas and skills to respond to the patient's needs.

   The need for a cultural paradigm shift is crucial. Simply replacing one model (say Roper, Logan and Tierney model) with the BNDU model will only frustrate practitioners who have been socialised to view the person from a functional perspective. Indeed, they will endeavour to continue to fit the patient to the model. As such, the foundation stone of the BNDU model is a vision for practice. I suspect few nurses would eschew holistic intent yet they are so locked into a functional approach they would be lost. Only through reflection can practitioners begin to feel the tension between the holistic ideal and their everyday practice.

9 Indeed this is essential work – see pages – regarding the absolute requirement of a valid vision for practice as the foundation stone for constructing and using the BNDU model.

10 The BNDU model is a reflexive form whereby it is continually tested and reformed in practice through systematic and structured reflection by its practitioners on its value to realise holistic practice. The whole notion of reflection is to gain insight that changes the practitioner and hence the practitioner's holistic practice is always in transition towards a more effective holistic practice that can only be known through reflection on practice. Holism in this sense is not merely an ideal but something only known through living it. Practitioners are always at different stages of 'knowing' holistic practice but this knowing is shared and co-created through group-guided reflection – see chapter 4.

REFERENCES

Ahmed L and Kitson A (1992) *The role of health care assistants within a professional nursing culture.* Institute of Nursing, Oxford.

Benner P (1984) *From novice to expert: excellence and power in clinical nursing practice.* Addison-Wesley, Menlo Park, California.

Benner P and Wrubel J (1989) *The primacy of caring: stress and coping in health and illness.* Addison-Wesley, Menlo Park, California.

Bond M (1984) *Pain: its nature, analysis and treatment.* Churchill Livingstone, Edinburgh.

Chin P and Jacobs M (1987) *Theory and nursing: a systematic approach* (second edition) C V. Mosby, St. Louis.

Egan G (1990) *The skilled helper: a systematic approach to effective helping.* Brooks/Cole Publishing, California.

Forster M (1989) *Have the men had enough?* Chatto and Windus, London.

Hockey L (1991) Foreword. In *Nursing as a therapy* (Eds. R McMahon and A Pearson) Chapman and Hall, London.

Hosking J and Welchew E (1985) *Post-operative pain: understanding its nature and how to treat it.* Faber and Faber, London.

Johns C (1990) Autonomy of primary nurses: the need to both facilitate and limit autonomy in practice. *Journal of Advanced Nursing* 15; 886–94.

Johns C (1991) The Burford nursing development unit holistic model of nursing practice. *Journal of Advanced Nursing* 16; 1090–8.

Kristjanson L, Tamblyn R, and Kuypers J (1987) A model to guide development and application of multiple nursing theories. *Journal of Advanced Nursing* 12; 523–9.

McCormack B (1992) Intuition: concept analysis and application to curriculum development. part 1. *Journal of Clinical Nursing* 1; 339–44.

McCormack B (1993) Intuition: concept analysis and application to curriculum development. part 2. *Journal of Clinical Nursing* 2; 11–7.

Meleis A (1991) *Theoretical nursing: development and progress.* Lippincott Company, Philadelphia.

Melia K (1990) (opposing the notion) Clinical nursing debates 1990 –nursing models: enhancing or inhibiting practice? *Nursing Standard* 5(11); 34–40.

Miller V and Rew L (1989) Analysis and intuition: the need for both in nurse education. *Journal of Nursing Education* 28(2); 84–6.

Mullooly V, Levin A, and Feldman H (1988) Music soothes post-operative pain and anxiety. *Journal of New York State Nurses Association* 19(3); 4–7.

National Health Service Health Advisory Services Department of Health and Social Services Inspectorate (1991) *Report on services for mentally ill people and elderly people in the Oxfordshire health district.* HAS/SSI(91)MI/E.63. HMSO, London.

Neuman B (1980) The Betty Neuman health care systems model: A total person approach to patient problems. In J P Riehl & C Roy (Ed.), *Conceptual models for nursing practice* (2nd ed., pp. 119–134). Appleton-Century-Crofts, New York.

Orem D (1980) *Nursing concepts of practice.* McGraw-Hill, New York.

Pyles S and Stern P (1983) Discovery of nursing gestalt in critical care nursing: the importance of the gray gorilla syndrome. *Image: The Journal of Nursing Scholarship* 15(2); 51–7.

Robinson K (1990) Nursing models – the hidden costs. *Surgical Nurse* 11; 13.

Roper N, Logan W, and Tierney A (1980) *The elements of nursing*. Churchill Livingstone, Edinburgh.

Ross R and Benditt E (1962) Wound healing and collagen formation. *Journal of Cell Biology* 12; 531–3.

Roy C (1989) The roy adaption model; the definitive statement. In *Conceptual models for nursing practice* (Ed. J Riehl-Sisca) Appleton and Lange, California.

Schon D (1983) *The reflective practitioner*. Basic Books, New York.

Smith P (1992) *The emotional labour of nursing: its impact on interpersonal relations, management and the educational environment in nursing*. MacMillan Education, Basingstoke.

Thomas S (1989) Pain and wound management. *Community Outlook* 1; 11–15.

Tucker H (1987) *The role and function of community hospitals*. King's Fund, London.

Visintainer M (1986) The nature of knowledge and theory in nursing. *Image: The Journal of Nursing Scholarship* 18(2); 32–38.

Watson J (1985) *Nursing: the philosophy and science of caring*. Colorado Associated University Press, Boulder.

Young C (1987) Intuition and the nursing process. *Holistic Nursing Practice* 1(3); 52–62.

Using the BNDU Model in the Community

CHAPTER 12

Susan Metcalf and Christopher Johns

This chapter describes the beginning of evaluating the impact of the BNDU model on my practice as a district nurse. This influence has been profound and led to a reassertion of my beliefs and values concerning the nature of district nursing.

THE USE OF MODELS OF NURSING IN MY PRACTICE

The district nursing team of which I am a member comprises two district nurses, one district enrolled nurse, one newly qualified staff nurse and three part-time auxiliary nurses. We work in a rural area covering a practice population of approximately 16,000 with a current caseload of 150 patients.

In our practice, as well as other teams within the Community NHS Trust we have used both the Roper, Logan and Tierney model (1980) and Orem's self-care model (1980). We chose these models because they were the most familiar to us, the easiest to use, and most appropriate to our organisational system. For example, the Roper, Logan and Tierney model's activities of living are reflected in many of the questions asked on the nursing assessment form which we are required to complete for the FIP nurse management system computer information package.

However, on refection of its value, I perceive the Roper, Logan and Tierney model as focusing my attention on seeing the patient as a set of task to be done framed within the activities of living. This is a functional approach to assessment and practice in contrast with the values-driven approach advocated by the BNDU model which reflects our, as yet, unstated beliefs concerning our vision of our district nursing practice.

As a team, we reflected on our use of the Roper, Logan and Tierney model to guide our practice. Firstly, there is a demand to fill in all the boxes as evidence of completing an assessment. However, we realised that information gained from some of the boxes was not relevant for many of the patients I work with. My preference had therefore been to use Orem's model as I felt it reflected my perceived role in enabling the patient to self-care.

I find that both models are long-winded and complex and (being sensible) I only document the information needed when nursing intervention is required; otherwise much of the information would be irrelevant. However, I feel this is an unsatisfactory practice as it fails to give a good overall picture of the patient. What is required is a concise and relevant assessment and ensuing plan for nursing the patient without having to wade through an excess of

Holistic Practice in Healthcare: The Burford NDU Person-centred Model, Second Edition. Edited by Christopher Johns.

information. In other words, within our busy workload lives, pragmatism is an important consideration.

On reviewing the BNDU model, the reality of heavy caseloads emerges as a significant limiting factor to caring for the whole person. If my caseload for the day consists of seeing 25 patients, it is very easy and sometimes very necessary to merely focus on the task; whether giving an injection, applying a dressing or inserting a catheter or indeed any task. The focus of work can then easily become one of controlling the environment in order to get through the work. This leads to defensiveness on the part of the district nurse who knows this is not the desired scenario. So we tend to rationalise our task approach to patients in order to cope, to blame it on the system or even to delude ourselves that we do see and care for the whole person.

But why do we need to see an overall picture of the whole person? As a team we informally discussed our beliefs and values about our nursing. As yet, we have not yet developed our own vision for practice and know that we must explore this further. Indeed, exploring the potential of the BNDU model prompted this activity. As Johns (1991) highlights, the use of the BNDU model is dependent on our realisation of our collective beliefs and values about our district nursing. Johns argues that the sensible use of any model of nursing should be based on the compatibility between beliefs and values of practitioners with the beliefs stated in the model's vision.

I find that using the BNDU model prompts me to constantly reflect on my beliefs and values. As such, these become more and more the basis of my practice rather than a mere orientation to tasks to be accomplished. As an experienced district nurse I ask myself – 'Why do I need to write my beliefs and values down? Isn't it enough to know these intuitively? Surely I know what district nursing is?' Johns argues (1991) that in writing them down, such beliefs are discussed, clarified and agreed as a way to give direction and meaning to practice. This gives direction to new staff and ensures that different nurses who visit the patient approach and respond to the patient with consistent and congruent care.

We felt the BNDU vision for practice was compatible with our own beliefs, in particular the espoused holistic approach that recognises and values the whole person.[1]

For example, when I apply a dressing the quality of care is related to my seeing the whole person, the person behind the dressing. Anything less than this is to treat the person with disrespect. Or in fact not to see the person at all but rather as some object I am doing something to. Such is the perversity of task-focused nursing. It is not enough to focus merely on the dressing or delight in my technical mastery in applying it while I subconsciously manipulate the environment to achieve my anticipated exit or more truthfully, to 'make my escape'. I say 'subconsciously' because admitting this fact to myself becomes unacceptable even as I rationalise this action in utilitarian terms of the needs of other patients needing my time.

As a consequence of adopting a holistic approach I have become more conscious of 'who I am' and my actions in response to the patient/person I am working with. (Even using the term 'person' rather than 'patient' gives greater recognition to their humanness as it does to myself). This results in a conscious shift from a position of manipulating the environment to one of dialogue and negotiation with the person. This does not mean I give them control but it recognises the essential worth of 'working with' the person. Obviously factors such as pressure to visit other patients, attend meetings, etc., influence this negotiation but patients know and respect that. It does not require defensive posturing. This fundamental shift from manipulation to negotiation is a shift from dishonesty that underpins all manipulation. As a consequence I no longer feel guilty and am more satisfied about doing a good job – indeed my workload stress is much reduced!

ANTICIPATORY VERSUS ADVERSARIAL ALLIANCES

As Johns notes in this book,[2] theory exists to inform practice and offers frameworks to view practice and gain insight. One particular theory I have found most helpful is the contrast between anticipatory and adversarial alliances (McLaughlin and Carey 1993). A negotiated relationship leads to an anticipatory alliance with the person. I use the word 'anticipatory' because negotiation is based on a mutual understanding of each other's expectations. As such, both my patients and myself are able to positively anticipate our planned meetings. In contrast I equate adversarial alliance with manipulation characterised by defensive manoeuvres that hinder open and honest communication necessary to achieve holistic practice. The patient can sense this and although they may say nothing, their body reflects the situation. The result is mutual discomfort that serves to strengthen the adversarial alliance. The visit becomes a suppressed conflict based on uncertainty, mismatched and unarticulated expectations, unmet needs and guardedness. The task is accomplished with compensatory glibness and contradictory words of reassurance and advice as we back towards the door anticipating our exit. Of course, much of this was below the radar as normal practice. It is reflecting on our beliefs that such previous normal ways of relating become apparent. Reflection is a wake-up blast!

The adversarial relationship is reminiscent of what Robinson and Thorne (1984) refer to as 'guarded alliance' between the nurse and the patient/relative in an attempt to reconstitute a relationship based on minimal conflict where at least some of the relatives' needs are met. The outcome is a blunting of the sensitivity of human caring and a process of mutual diminishment. Both the nurse and the patient are impoverished in the process and both feel less than satisfied by the encounter. In contrast, anticipatory alliance is akin to what Robinson and Thorne note as 'naïve trusting' whereby the patient/family believe that the caring staff view the situation from their perspective and have their best interests at heart. As I will show later in the chapter, the BNDU model naturally guides the practitioner to appreciating such perspective. When the patient realises the caring staff view the situation differently it leads to disenchantment, conflict and breakdown of communication. Of course, this is unsatisfactory leading the patient to reconstruct the relationship, albeit cautiously to form a guarded alliance.

Seeing my relationships through these theoretical frameworks has been eye opening.

RESPECTING GUESTS

Obviously, the external environment of practice at Burford is different from the environment of care in our district nursing practice, with the patient being nursed in their own home rather than in a hospital setting. Away from the depersonalising environment of the hospital, it is more likely that we are able to see the 'whole' person. It is important we respect the person as we are guests in their home. It is equally important we respect patients as people in hospital. The difference is that within the home we are 'invited guests' whereas in hospital the patient is the 'invited guest'.

Reflecting on the different environments of care, led us to change two of the BNDU reflective cues to reflect this:

1. 'What health event brings this person into hospital?' became 'What health event prompts my visit to this person?'

2. 'What is important for this person to make their stay in hospital comfortable?' became 'What is important for the person to make my visit comfortable for them?' Otherwise we felt in tune with the BNDU cues.[3]

REFLECTIONS ON THE USE OF THE BNDU MODEL

On a superficial level we found the BNDU model simple to use and instinctively felt it was useful tool to assessing the patient. The enrolled nurse and myself thought that the cues were actually what we tended to think of when assessing a patient. In this respect the BNDU model reflects a natural process of our caring rather than asking us to interpret the way we perceive a patient into more complex and alien patterns which the Roper, Logan and Tierney and Orem models inclined us to do. In this way the BNDU assessment cues made us both feel more competent and confident in our assessment of patients.

The newly qualified staff nurse found the cues very helpful as she had little experience in assessment. What experience she had had was hospital focused using models of nursing that she said had little personal meaning to her. From a philosophical perspective, this concept of *personal meaning* is an important consideration in using a model of nursing. I feel that a model of nursing needs to become an extension of the nurse as a natural way to relating appropriately to the person. In other words, it becomes a part of who I am – not a tool to apply.

By using the BNDU model, our assessments now give a much better overall picture of the patient and clearly lead to recognising and selecting appropriate interventions to meet the patient's and family's needs, and for many dependent patients, the support to remain in their own homes. We feel our care planning has improved and we now pay more attention to the patient's psycho-social need, and recognise and understand the impact of our feelings towards the patient in considering how best to help the patients meet these needs.

We shall illustrate the use of the BNDU model in practice through 3 case studies.

PATSY: A DIFFICULT PATIENT?

Patsy was referred to our district nursing team by social services for a 'help bath'. She was known to me as we had visited her to give enemas and dietary advice during episodes of constipation. I had only met Patsy a couple of times as she was my colleague's patient.

She was well known for being a 'difficult' patient and a 'troublemaker'. An article had appeared in the local paper about her not getting enough help as she was housebound. We felt this was very unfair as she was receiving daily homecare. She had also been offered respite care that she had cancelled at the last minute. The article gave the impressions that she was a very neglected old lady. I felt very negative towards her as I knew her reputation and feelings of my colleagues, home-carers and the general practitioner.

When I visited her I found that she was very lonely, she had never married and her only relative was a nephew who lived 40 miles away so she did not see him often. She used to be the local district nurse so she had preconceived ideas about her care. She could not understand that 'times had changed' and she kept saying 'it was not like this in my day'. She felt that she had got the 'short straw'. She would have really liked to go into a residential care home but she did not see why she should have to use her 'hard earned' savings to contribute to her care.

By using the BNDU cues – 'how must this person be feeling?', 'How does this person make me feel?' and 'How does this person view the future?' I gave much more thought trying to understand Patsy and could talk with her about her feelings and thoughts for the future. It made me conscious of how important it was for me and my colleagues to be aware of our feelings towards this person in order to be able to understand why she was behaving in that way that led us to originally perceive her as 'difficult' and which led me to visit her with preconceived ideas based on that label.

Using the cue questions guided me to explore with Patsy the reasons for her behaviour. As a consequence I could accept this lady for who she was and could understand how she felt about her predicament. Visiting to give her a bath only reinforced her sense of helplessness and loss of control. She needed to be understood and in control of her future.

As a result, she responded much more positively towards me, coming to trust me as someone who was genuinely concerned for her rather than as someone to fight against. This experience was a salutary lesson of the perversity of labelling someone as 'difficult' and how this leads nurses and others to picture a person in such negative terms. I felt very positive towards Patsy as a result of my visits to her. What I originally perceived as a threatening and stressful encounter became an enlightening and satisfying experience. Yet I ask myself – 'why did it take such a simple cue question to fundamentally reorientate my practice?' I can only draw the conclusion of how blind to caring we can become due to trying to cope with pressures of work. This again reminds me of what Johns (1991) describes as the 'internal environment' – one in which practitioners relate to each other in ways that allow the patient to be valued as a person despite the difficulties that sometimes creates. Recognising that we do value the whole person makes it essential we address this issue in our practice. Otherwise we risk leading contradictory lives where our values and practice are incompatible and we hide behind our rationalisations to protect ourselves.[4]

ANNIE

This second case study is focused around introducing the BNDU model to my student district nurse. Her initial reaction was that several visits would have to be made to a patient before an assessment could be completed from which a care plan could be drawn up for the patient. She was not convinced that by using the BNDU model we would have enough information for such action. However, she was willing to try it.

We visited the patient who was referred to us by the Oncology clinic the previous day for dressings to a fungating breast tumour. The student used the BNDU assessment cues to frame her assessment.

WHO IS THIS PERSON?

Annie is an 86-year-old lady who has been widowed for a few years. She has one daughter and two grandchildren. Her only sister died six months ago of breast carcinoma. She has recently moved into a 'granny annexe' in her daughter's home. She says she doesn't really miss where she used to live as she hadn't many friends there anyway.

WHAT HEALTH EVENT HAD PROMPTED MY VISIT TO THIS PERSON?

She was referred to use from the Oncology clinic to assess her needs and redress a fungating breast carcinoma. Annie told us that she first noticed discharge from her breast about 6 years ago but she hoped it would go away and anyways she was far too busy looking after her husband and then her sister to bother about it. Once she had moved into her new flat, her daughter noticed it and immediately took her to the GP. He immediately referred her on to the Oncology clinic but did not refer her to us as the daughter said she was quite happy to redress the wound. The Oncology clinics were not happy with the dressings and felt that Annie would benefit from having us visit.

HOW MUST THIS PERSON BE FEELING?

She appears to be fairly cheerful and says she doesn't want to be a bother.

HOW HAS THIS EVENT AFFECTED HER USUAL LIFE PATTERN AND ROLES?

It doesn't appear to be affecting her life pattern at present, apart from requiring regular visits from us. She says she likes being at home and at the moment does not want to go out and socialise. In her previous home she said that neither she or her husband went out much.

HOW DOES THIS PERSON MAKE ME FEEL?

On first impression she is very pleasant likeable old lady. I feel sad that she was not referred to us earlier as we could have made her feel much more comfortable with a more appropriate dressing.

HOW CAN I HELP THIS PERSON?

By redressing her breast as appropriate to make her feel comfortable. I can also refer her to other agencies as required and give support to her and her family.

WHAT IS IMPORTANT FOR THIS PERSON TO MAKE MY VISIT COMFORTABLE FOR HER?

This is difficult to answer after only one visit. Annie said she would be pleased to see us at any time – whatever suited us best.

WHAT SUPPORT DOES THIS PERSON HAVE?

Annie lives in close proximity with her daughter and family. It means that family are around her when she needs them, but she can also continue to lead an independent life. She is able to do her household chores with the help of a weekly private cleaner. She cooks for herself but joins the family for Sunday lunch. Her daughter shops for her, but Annie is able to walk to the local shop. We shall be visiting daily to redress her breast.

HOW DOES SHE VIEW THE FUTURE FOR HERSELF AND OTHERS?

On first impression Annie does not seem to be looking a long way into the future. She is waiting to go into hospital for a mastectomy that she is dreading. She says she will be glad when it is all over and she's back at home.

From this initial assessment that only took 45 minutes, we were able to draw up a care plan which, on our next visit, we showed Annie and asked if she agreed or wanted to add anything. The student was surprised at the detail obtained after just one visit and the simplicity of the model to use.

She felt that some cues were difficult to answer, for example – 'How must this person be feeling?' and 'How does this person make me feel?' and 'What is important for this person to make my visit comfortable for her?' Yet we both felt better, more satisfied, having acknowledged both Annie's and own feelings. Without doubt we felt that this acknowledgement was essential in developing a relationship with Annie and the information we had obtained could be built on through future visits.

I find it difficult to write negative feelings about a person and impossible to actually tell them that I don't like them. Yet I believe I should show a patient what I have written about them not least because the notes are left with the person. I know of course that the cues are simply that – cues – and do not need concrete answers. I know that but it highlights my difficulty using the model with the way I have been socialised into using models in a passive and deterministic way, notably that boxes are meant to be filled in! Nurses need to be intelligent in using the BNDU model, to see it as a tool to enable them to realise effective holistic practice rather than a task in itself that needs completing. When I feel negative about a patient I need to understand why and deal with it so it does not interfere with being available to the person – to turn that negative feeling or energy into positive energy and action.

Returning to Patsy's case study I wrote in her notes (narrative) –

> *Patsy feels lonely and anxious about the cost of moving into residential care. Our aim is to understand how she feels about her present situation and the future and to help her make the best decision.*

In this way, I channelled my negative feelings into a positive channel. I also helped my colleagues deal with their own negative feelings towards Patsy. Building up a positive therapeutic relationship and plan of care developed over future visits for both Patsy and Annie, as indeed with all our patients, as if a work in progress. No longer patients are seen as 'difficult' but as suffering, struggling human beings needing some help.

CONNIE

My third case study is a reflection on my first experience of using the BNDU model to reassess a patient I had been nursing for 4 years. Although I realised that the cues were designed to tune me into my holistic beliefs I used the cues to structure the assessment (rather like my student nurse did in the previous case study). I felt this necessary to 'get to know the cues' as the BNDU approach seemed alien in comparison with my previous experiences using the Roper, Logan and Tierney and Orem models.[5]

WHO IS THIS PERSON?

Connie is 74 years old and lives alone in a council-owned bungalow. She has three living children. One son died in a road traffic accident many years ago. One daughter lives in Australia and she writes regularly. Her son also lives locally but he does not visit his mother often.

HOW MUST THIS PERSON BE FEELING?

Connie says she feels 'useless' and hates having to rely on others to help her with personal and household tasks. She does get tearful at times and anxious if she is unwell as she does not want to be admitted to hospital again. Her husband left home 6 months ago following a family argument. She is very upset as they had been married for 54 years. However, she has since confided that the marriage had not been a happy one. She says that in a way she is relieved that he has left although 'it is still upsetting after all those years together'. Now she is worried in case he walks in, as she insists she does not want him back. She is having to get used to living alone but she says it has not been too difficult as he was out for much of the day and evening. She doesn't feel lonely as her neighbours, friends and daughter are visiting her more often now.

HOW HAS THIS HEALTH EVENT AFFECTED HER NORMAL LIFE PATTERN AND ROLES?

Over the years Connie has adapted to being in a wheelchair. She now has a microwave oven that has enabled her to cook, as she was finding it too difficult using a conventional oven. This has helped her a lot as her husband used to lift heavy saucepans on and off the cooker. She can also manage simple household tasks such as dusting and ironing which she does enjoy doing and says she has always been house-proud.

Her home has been adapted to meet some of her needs, for example, a raised toilet seat and frame and a monkey pole and bedlocks that help her get in and out of bed more easily. She is now unable to go out without help but says she is happy to stay at home. She cannot get into a car now so her outings are restricted to local walks and to her daughter's home.

She has only recently been able to do this as she has a urinary catheter in situ. At first when she had the catheter she wasn't very keen but now she is delighted as it has given her freedom to go out, whereas before she could only use the toilet at her home.

HOW CAN I HELP THIS PERSON?

I can help Connie by listening to her problems and advising her I visit weekly to help her wash and dress and to check that her pressure sores are intact and give catheter care.

WHAT IS IMPORTANT FOR THIS PERSON TO MAKE MY VISIT COMFORTABLE FOR HER?

Connie likes to know which member of the team is going to visit. She likes her visit as near to 09.00 as possible. As she does not like being in her night clothes in her wheelchair. She realises that this may not possible every visit as we may have to see other patients early. We always let her know approximately what time we will visit and she always appreciates this.

WHAT SUPPORT DOES THIS PERSON HAVE?

Connie received a lot of help from the district nurses, social services, family and friends. She is visited daily by either the district nurse team or by home-carers. We alternate to help Connie wash and dress daily. Home-care also gives her an hour a week to clean the bungalow and change her bedding. Her friends and neighbour help her with the washing and any other jobs that home-care may not have time to do, such as cleaning the windows.

Her daughter does all her shopping and also prepares some meals for. Connie goes every Sunday to her daughter's home. She always contacts her daily by phone or personally to ensure Connie is comfortable and has everything she needs. Connie is always appreciative of this care as her daughter also works and says she has her own life to lead.

HOW DOES SHE VIEW THE FUTURE FOR HERSELF AND FOR OTHERS?

Connie is concerned about the future. She says that she wonders what will happen to her when she can no longer transfer from bed to wheelchair. She wants to stay in her own home, but if ever the time comes when she cannot look after herself she does not want to go into residential care. She has discussed this with her daughters and they have both said they would look after her in their own homes. She is relieved about this but says she doesn't want to burden them.

Over a period of time it is easy to take for granted aspects of a patient's care and to become complacent about one's helping role. Connie's case study illustrates the ease with which I used the BNDU model. The cues helped me review Connie's total care and putting it down as a narrative on paper made the information available to my colleagues, enabling them to see Connie as I saw her. However, it may take us all some time to adjust to writing in this 'narrative style'. Yet, it does paint a valuable whole picture.

It is interesting to reflect on the cue 'How has this event affected the person's normal life pattern and roles'. Thinking about Roper, Logan and Tierney's activities of living I would look at the issues surrounding these: mobility, eating, sleeping, eliminating, working and playing that complement each other. Initially I did wonder if the BNDU cues would give a detailed enough assessment. My fears were unfounded. Rather than these issues being discrete activities they now merged into a 'wholeness' that made immediate sense! The wholeness was maintained throughout our visits and yet the detail remained. Neither the Roper, Logan and Tierney model or the Orem model encouraged us to see Connie from a holistic perspective, notably psychosocial aspects of care. The emphasis on universal self-care requisites and activities of living is physically oriented. Also the wording of Orem's more psychosocial self-care requisites are difficult to interpret.

ORGANISATIONAL CONSEQUENCES OF USING THE BNDU MODEL

Using the BNDU model prompted a review of the amount and relevance of material demanded by the FIP computer system.[6] In this sense the BNDU is empowering because its reflective nature encouraged the team to challenge and take control of our practice in a positive rather than reactive or defensive way.

The BNDU model certainly helped us to reflect on our beliefs and values regarding the core nature of district nursing. This is significant not just in the sense of patient care. It relates to what Johns (1991) describes as the 'external environment of care' in questioning the purpose of district nursing and its organisational context that has radically changed with the advent of GP fundholding and NHS Trusts. In this changing climate district nurses must assert the nature of their role.

With the implementation of the Community Care Act (1990) there have been changes affecting the way in which we give care in the community. A pilot project was undertaken to look into care management and one of its conclusions was the need for good assessment of the patient by an assessor who was not connected to either health or social services. There was also a need for shared documentation to prevent duplication of information. I discussed the potential of the BNDU model with the pilot project coordinator for use as the basis for assessment. We both felt we needed to pursue this idea as the BNDU model seemed an ideal model as a multi-disciplinary approach.

CONCLUSIONS

As a team I realise we need a vision for our practice. We have discussed the Burford hospital vision and we feel in tune with it, but feel it does need some adapting for our environment of practice. I hope that our district nursing group will do this and, as a result, more nurses will use the BNDU model.

At present, we keep the completed assessments rather than leaving them with patients in their own homes. This has proved to be very helpful, particularly when visiting a patient for the first time as an associate nurse as the assessments give a good overall picture of the patient. They have been written concisely and are easy to read, giving the relevant information to effectively continue and adapt care as necessary.

Inevitably the work described in this chapter can only give partial attention to the development of the BNDU model in our district nursing practice. It is difficult to explain how such a seemingly simple model can re-nurture such a sense of commitment in me towards nursing. It has enabled and empowered me to at once voice, value and enact my caring beliefs. And it is not just me. The model is viewed with considerable hope and optimism by my colleagues as a framework for guiding practice. Over time, environmental factors have a limiting effect on caring practice; thus it has been important to refocus the meaning of district nursing practice.

The ideas in this chapter are a reflection of my dialogue with Christopher Johns helping me to make sense of the model. He felt it was important I make this contribution because so often such books are written by theorists rather than by ordinary practitioners reflecting on their struggle to make sense of their practice and emergent theory. I have never been critical before of either my practice or theory. Though aware of the coming and going of theories I had taken refuge in my habitualised practice. I make this point in order to give courage to other practitioners who feel oppressed by or shelter from reflection on their practice. We all have a responsibility to develop our practice in order to meet the needs of our patients more effectively assuming that nurses do want to care for their patients. Embracing the BNDU model may seem simple but in reality it is a massive culture shift where old norms must be confronted and new ways of being established.

Without doubt, to embrace the BNDU model is to embrace holistic caring as the core of nursing, an embrace that opens the door to mutual ways of working with patients and mutual satisfaction within our caring relationships. In this way we are all winners!

NOTES

1 Articulating one's beliefs and values is not necessarily an easy thing to do – simply because practitioners have not been asked to do this before. Even a notion of what a 'belief' is may be difficult to answer. Hence, reading another vision may help practitioners from other settings to get an idea of what a vision looks like – and whether they agree with it. This is a first step. Later, it can be reflected on and refined to suit the particular setting. Here we see the value of the Burford vision to challenge and confront others.

2 For many practitioners theory is outside their frame of reference to practice. They simply are not exposed to it despite many available nursing journals. They just get on with the job, leaving theoretical production and debate to academics often far removed from actual practice, dipping into it to carry out research. Hence there has been this much vaunted theory-practice gap. Sue became exposed to the theories cited through dialogue in guided reflection with myself as practical ways to frame her shift towards holistic relationships with patients rather than task-focused relationships. The theories made sense and became internalised within her practical knowing. This juxtaposition of theoretical knowledge with practical knowing is related to the deepening insights phase of reflection within the Model for Structured Reflection (see Appendix 1).

3 Any practice considering adopting the BNDU model will necessarily match their beliefs and values to the Burford vision because the cues emanate from the vision as the way to tune the practitioner into the vision when throughout their practice. The district nurses felt in tune with the Burford vision, prompting them to realise the need to construct their own vision. One difficulty they face is being 'captured' by the language of the Burford vision that is compelling and speaks in a practical language for anyone who aspires to holistic practice.

4 Sue illustrates how adopting a holistic approach actually eases stress because it enabled her to be herself and respond to Patsy with her humanely rather than as some difficult object to deal with. As a result, Sue felt liberated, free from stress and discovered that her holistic approach led to more mean-

ingful and satisfying work – in other words reconnected to caring is a major stress buster whereas leading contradictory lives emerges as a major stress inducer.

Sue reinforces the idea of creating the therapeutic team (as evidenced in other accounts in the book) to ensure a consistent approach and support each other. As team leader she saw this as her responsibility, reinforcing her concept of self as a team leader.

5 It remained to be seen whether Susan was able to influence the current nursing input into the organisational FIP computer system. Her comments highlight how such systems reduce practitioners to 'slaves'; imputing useless information without any benefit, as if to say, 'we have invested in this technology and you will use it regardless'. In busy lives practitioners need tools that are useful to record and communicate information. Yet as Susan alludes – the BNDU model has enabled her to find a political voice to take action and begin to shift the external environment to support holistic practice through the use of the BNDU model.

REFERENCES

DHSS (1990) National health service and community care act. HMSO, London.

Johns C (1991) The Burford nursing development unit holistic model of nursing practice. *Journal of Advanced Nursing* 16; 1090–8.

McLaughlin A M and Carey J L (1993) The adversarial relationship: developing therapeutic relationships between families and the team in brain injury rehabilitation. *Brain Injury* 7(1); 45–59.

Orem D E (1980) *Nursing concepts of practice*. McGraw-hill Book Company, New York.

Robinson C A and Thorne S E (1984) Strengthening patient interference. *Journal of Advanced Nursing* 9; 597–602.

Roper N, Logan W W, and Tierney A (1980) *The elements of nursing*. Churchill Livingstone, Edinburgh.

Applying the BNDU Model in an Acute Medical Unit [7e]

CHAPTER 13

Robert Garbett

This chapter is an account of practitioners considering the use of the BNDU model as a framework for practice in an acute medical unit. The nursing team on 7e have progressed from a medical model orientation to considering the potential of nursing as an independent therapeutic agent as well as an inter-dependent part of hospital health care. Primary nursing has been adopted as an organisational vehicle for nursing work and has been adapted to suit the demands of acute nursing where the average length of stay is 5 days.

USING MODELS IN PRACTICE

Generally speaking, nursing models have been deductively derived from extant theory from the natural and social sciences. Various nurse theorists (for example Roy (Roy and Andrews 1991) and Orem (1991)) mention that their own practice influenced their work but there is little evidence to suggest that the most popularly adopted models have been derived inductively from the experience of practice.

Whilst the various models of nursing may have something to offer nursing practice, and there exists no conclusive proof that they do (Chapman 1990).The world of practice erects a number of barriers between the idealisation and practice of nursing (Miller 1985). Nursing models have been adopted without question, instead of as a tool to be used critically (Gordon 1984, Lister 1987). It has been suggested that for practicing nurses the adoption of nursing models has proved restrictive rather than facilitative to practice (Gordon 1984). Another frequently cited barrier to the use of models is that of the use of difficult language in describing concepts within them (Gordon 1984, Gruending 1985, Miller 1985). Nurses in the UK using models originating in USA have discovered that such models are in some ways culturally inappropriate to practice in the UK (Wright 1989, Draper 1990).

On 7e, Orem's self-care deficit model was adopted because it most closely matched the views of the ward team as contained in the ward philosophy at that time. Since then, current members of the ward team have been asked for their views about various nursing process issues including some questions about the use of models. The majority of the team named Orem as the model used in the ward. However, the extent to which this meant the strategy or the concepts of 'self-care deficit' underlying the model is unclear, from such expressions as 'I use a vague interpretation of Orem's', it seemed that it was more than the former than the latter. It seemed that there was a ground swell of independent practice with individuals adapting their approach and suggesting that using the model was rigid and restrictive. Previously

Holistic Practice in Healthcare: The Burford NDU Person-centred Model, Second Edition. Edited by Christopher Johns.

adopted beliefs were still influential, especially with regard to thinking around 'helping patients care for themselves'.

Partly because Orem as a model is now considered inadequate to frame practice, a period of re-evaluation is now taking place on the ward with the BNDU model as one possible contribution.

THE WARD PHILOSOPHY

Several years after the initial development work on 7e, there was once again a need to revisit the conceptual basis underpinning practice. Since decisions were made about philosophical beliefs and suitable theoretical strategies there had been a substantial turnover of staff.

The BNDU model is founded on Burford hospital's philosophy. A preliminary step to establishing the model's suitability for adoption on 7e is therefore the examination of our ward philosophy vis a vis that of Burford.

Only 4 members out of 20 survive from when the existing ward philosophy was written in 1990 and, as such, was due for review in light of changes of personnel and different influences (Johns 1991). The existing philosophy had been reviewed on two previous occasions and agreed as adequate. This 'adequacy' can be challenged:

- Is the philosophy still an integral part of practitioners' thinking?
- Is the notion of a ward philosophy perceived as relevant to practice or just a conceptual nicety?
- Is it seen as a subject worth spending time and energy on?

The revised philosophy (Figure 13.1) is analysed using the key components of a philosophy identified by Johns (1989):

- External environment of care
- Internal environment of care
- Social viability
- The nature of care[1]

EXTERNAL ENVIRONMENT OF CARE

At present, notions of environmental factors that enable as well as constrain the provision of nursing care are not contained within the philosophy. However, there are factors within the external environment that do have a bearing on care provided by the ward. Recognition of such factors is important if the philosophy is to be used as a document that 'attempts to capture the tension between the reality of practice and beliefs and values of its practitioners' (Johns 1991).

The Oxford Radcliffe hospital provides emergency services for a wide geographical area. It works with a network of more specialised centres and a number of community hospitals. Nurses within the hospital can expect to work within a complex web of other professionals both within and outside hospital.

This is a statement of some of our shared values and beliefs that guide our nursing practice on 7e.

Every patient deserves the unconditional warm regard of the nurses. Every person is a unique individual with social, psychological, spiritual and physical needs who should be allowed to make informed choices which the nurses will respect. If it seems appropriate, the nurses will encourage family and friends to be closely involved in the patient's care.

To us, the most important aspect of nursing is caring. This includes the development of a partnership between the nurse and the patient. The aim of the partnership is to meet the patient's needs but at the same time foster personal control and the growth of independence.

Nursing care is provided by a team of nurses, each with a valuable and unique contribution to make. We acknowledge the importance of continuity of care and endeavour to provide this to our patients by using a primary nursing system. On admission every patient is assigned to a small team of nurses, one of whom will be the named primary nurse. The primary nurse will be responsible for the planning of care with the patient using a systematic approach.

Whenever on duty, the primary nurse will look after the patient. In his/her absence, the associate nurse(s) will continue care as planned. Any unqualified member of staff will be supervised by a qualified member of the nursing team.

Knowledge enables people to look after themselves and helps prevent reoccurrence or exacerbation of illness. It is therefore an important nursing responsibility to educate patients and their families.

Nurses are part of a multi-disciplinary team which works together for the benefit of the patient. Success of this team depends on cooperation and good communication.

Nursing care is prescribed using up-to-date nursing knowledge and in the light of experience. It is every nurse's responsibility to continue his/her education and share this knowledge with others. Learning opportunities are provided on the ward and staff are encouraged to attend study days whenever possible.

FIGURE 13.1 7e ward philosophy (second edition)

The medical wards fulfil a number of functions, some or all of which may be carried out in providing nursing to an individual:

- The assessment and support of an acutely ill patient
- Complementing and supporting medical interventions
- The initiation and provision of rehabilitation
- Discharge planning
- Health education
- The provision of palliative care when a person is dying

Any philosophical underpinning and nursing model would need to reflect this broad range of activity and the approach to working which are responsive to the needs of both long- and short-stay patients who are experiencing a wide range of problems.

The 7e philosophy could therefore be developed more in relation to exploring tensions between practical constraints and ideological aspirations. At present, the philosophy focused principally on the nurse-patient relationship whilst acknowledging the potential for involvement of family and friends in a patient's care. The ward's status as a Nursing Development Unit places new responsibilities on it and these have yet to be expressed explicitly within the ward's philosophy. Such responsibilities are apparent in the Burford philosophy (see Figure 1.1) and the resultant model for practice. A fuller consideration of contextual issues related to the ward's position within and outside the Oxford Radcliffe hospital in future reformulation of the philosophy may help team members situate their work within a broader picture.

INTERNAL ENVIRONMENT

The internal environment is concerned with relationships between colleagues and other health professionals. The Burford philosophy (see Figure 1.1) and Johns's work on therapeutic teams (1992) describe the need for relationships between staff to be founded on similar holistic principles to those between practitioners and patients. This focus is contained within our philosophy to a certain extent. The lived experience of working on the ward suggests that nurses adopt similar attitudes to each other as they do with patients, if anecdotal comments of those who work on the ward are to be believed. Similar support systems as described at Burford are well established. Regular review of performance takes place, albeit informally at times. Regular meetings are held to discuss ward progress. Various forms of personal and professional development are actively encouraged and supported through an agreed minimum of study leave per year.[2] The devising and refinement of flexible work patterns has been defined and is under constant review so that team members may optimise their contribution to the ward as a whole while following other paths in their lives (for instance, having a family or becoming a full-time student).

Environmental constraints are most apparent when considering the philosophy statements concerning the manner in which care delivery is organised:

> *We acknowledge the importance of continuity of care and endeavour to provide this for our patients by using a primary nursing system. On admission a patient is allocated to a small team of nurses, one of whom will be the named primary nurse.*

However, this does not always happen. The continuity demanded by this statement requires a degree of organisational complexity, which, with the demands placed by annual leave, days off, and study days becomes difficult to the extent where continuity cannot always be afforded. This difficulty is compounded by the high turnover of patients. In effect this means that many of the people that nurses meet stay for only 24–48 hours. Some stay for a number of weeks or even months. As a result, the approaches nurses utilise conceptually and in their records need to be flexible to meet widely varying paces of work.

The opinions of the ward team elicited so far would indicate that at present this is not necessarily the case. The number of comments concerning how much time is consumed in recording assessments and care plans for patients would seem to indicate, along with the patchy nature of records reviewed from patients' notes, that the means of satisfactorily representing nursing thoughts and actions have not yet been found. This applies particularly to patients whose stay in hospital is relatively short. The pressures placed on the continuity of care by the members of the nursing team put great demand on their communication skills. Arguably, such a degree of task complexity requires clarity when it comes to outlining the responsibility of nurses both individually and collectively. At present this clarity is lacking from the philosophy statement –

This primary nurse will be responsible for the planning of care... using a systematic approach.

Especially so in the light of team members holding differing views as to the merits and content of such a 'systematic approach'.

The organisation of the ward's nursing team reflects beliefs influenced by the development of responsibility. The work on supportive hierarchies (Ryan 1989) has been influential. A support hierarchy has as its objective quality care for its clients wherein control of events is ideally invested in the client. The provider of the service (the practitioner) is accountable to the client and is supported by senior colleagues who act as resources and facilitators, as well as educators, associates, learners and ancillary staff. The practitioner works in collaboration with other members of the multi-disciplinary team. In effect, the pyramidal nature of a hierarchy, with leaders on top and workers to the base, is turned on its head.[3] The resources of the organisation are employed to support the practitioners in their encounters with clients.

On 7e, a system of collective decision-making has evolved. The ward is led by a group of senior practitioners who support the team as a whole. Administrative tasks that have traditionally been the domain of the ward sister are devolved throughout the team and rotated on a regular basis. It can be said therefore, that in terms of what happens on the ward there is a strong relationship between the nature of nurse-patient relationships and those between nurses themselves. Relationships are oriented towards affording development of, and opportunity for, individual responsibility.

May (1992), in a qualitative study involving the observation of 22 staff nurses in Scotland, speaks of patients being given 'multiple and disconnected identities' by the various staff that they encounter during their hospital stay. In a busy teaching hospital such as the Oxford Radcliffe, the majority of occupational groups involved in the day-to-day care of patients are subject to relatively high turnover. House Officers may work on a ward between 2 and 6 months, senior house officers only slightly longer. Physiotherapists, dieticians, and occupational therapists move every 4 months. Nurses who usually work for at least a year if not considerably longer in one practice setting provide constancy.

Writing from the perspective of a nurse who has seen medical and paramedical staff pass through my own clinical area, the notion of patients being given 'multiple and disconnected identities' is persuasive. Conflict may occasionally arise. Whilst such conflicts may be productively resolved through negotiation, a situation where there is a consistent and unified multi-disciplinary approach for any length of time is difficult to achieve. The articulation of a nursing philosophy is a recent phenomenon and seems to have a unifying influence of nursing staff when they have been involved in the writing on the way they work and relate to each other.

SOCIAL VIABILITY

As described by Johns (1991) the concept of social viability is adopted from the work of Dorothy Johnson (1974). While, arguably, the 7e philosophy is incomplete,[4] it reflects a degree of social significance. Its contents are shared with patients usually at an early stage of their stay.

Within environments where public expectations are 'to toe the line' when in hospital (Waterworth and Luker 1990), notions of active participation in their own care may seem alien to patients. However, with support from their nurses, patients can journey from feeling that they have to conform to a set of expectations to a point where they can express themselves more freely. This is an area of the ward philosophy that can possibly be evaluated.

Political statements are implicit within the 7e philosophy, in particular the belief that in an acute setting patients deserve the care of a professional nurse. This belief is underpinned by the beliefs of nursing leaders, such as Pembrey (1984) and by more recent work examining the relative merits of differing skill and grade mixes. Work on skill mix has examined the 'value for money' of care delivered by qualified nurses (Hancock 1992). She cites studies such as that by Helt and Jellinek (1988) in arguing that a high ratio of qualified nurses has the potential to increase efficiency. The study 'Ward nursing quality and grade mix' (Bagust et al. 1992) suggested that in some settings a smaller work force with higher proportion of qualified nurses delivers higher quality of patient care and is more cost effective.

THE NATURE OF CARE

According to the 7e philosophy, caring is the most important aspect of nursing. Although the exact nature of caring is not articulated, components of caring are implicit within it. These include:

- The development of a partnership between nurse and patient with the partnership orientated towards both meeting the person's needs while fostering personal growth and control.
- The provision of knowledge to avoid future reoccurrence or exacerbation of illness.

Stress is laid on the importance of the use of up-to-date knowledge as well as experience in the prescription of nursing care.

The influence of these concepts from within humanism and phenomenology described by Johns (1991) are apparent, in particular, the notion of working with patients towards their improved health through considering social, psychological, spiritual and physical needs.

Given that the Burford model of nursing flows from philosophical concepts, it is a necessary first step to examine the congruity between these concepts and the philosophy developed on 7e in considering the suitability of the model for adaption to an acute medical setting. The external environment of the two units is different to an extent. The difference lies in the greater complexity of relationships and speed of turnover on 7e. Nurses on 7e possibly meet patients at a different stage of their hospital career than at Burford. The internal environment is more explicitly examined within the Burford philosophy. However, initiatives on 7e exemplify staff relationships which parallel those we strive to offer patients.

The principle areas of congruence between the two philosophies are in dealing with nurse-patient and nurse-nurse relationships. An area of divergence is that of a more individualistic approach described within the 7e philosophy than that found within the Burford philosophy. However, the degree of divergence in practice is difficult to assess. Overall, it would seem that the philosophical approaches of both units have much in common and that the model arising from the Burford philosophy may be congruent with practice on 7e.

USING THE BNDU MODEL

Since reading Johns (1991) I have used ideas contained within the model in my practice. Similarly, colleagues have tried out the assessment strategy in particular. The immediate appeal of the model lies in the posing of the very simple and pragmatic question – 'what information do I need to nurse this patient?' It is this pragmatic approach that we frequently adopt as a response to an environment where the demands of workload fluctuate rapidly. As a result, the priorities in our work are primarily providing care and time required for completing nursing records is resented, especially where its content is perceived to be repetitive and irrelevant. Of 12 respondents to a questionnaire I gave 7e nurses, 8 identified paperwork as the most unpopular aspect of the nursing process. Six respondents also identified present practice as repetitive, for example – 'Do we really need to write at such lengths that which is of no relevance to us and which creates no problem or is of little or no relevance?'

The responses to my questionnaire support findings of a detailed qualitative study of 4 Canadian nurses (Howse and Bailey 1992). These authors describe what they term intrinsic and extrinsic factors which make documentation difficult for nurses. Intrinsic factors include difficulties with written expression and the feeling that 'doing it is more important than writing about it'. Extrinsic factors include the format of documents and the time required to complete them within busy and pressured work settings.

In the course of keeping in mind the strategy of the BNDU model while working with patients, I find it lends itself to flexible approaches of documenting issues of concern to colleagues. For example, the accepted practice of waiting for a relationship to form with a patient before formal assessment can mean that the amount of information available about patients can be small. Some of the ward team have adopted the practice of presenting an abbreviated sketch of the most prominent concerns about a patient to 'fill the gap' before a fuller assessment is presented. At times, this sketch can suffice for a patient is short stay or relatively uncomplicated.

For example, this summary was written about a middle-aged woman, Susan, when she was admitted for a suspected pulmonary embolus:

Areas of concern:
Married woman who has been unwell for 5 days, 'bad chest'
Pain – worse on inspiration, left lower chest, mainly at back
Productive cough with blood stained sputum
? pulmonary embolus, no apparent risk factors

While this summary could undoubtedly have been fuller, and as this person's stay in hospital went on, more complex areas of concern became apparent, it provided an answer to an immediate question of – 'what information do I need to nurse this patient?' From this base I could then, equally briefly, identify – 'How can I help this person?', framing both her and her family's concerns – fear, uncertainty and pain – with those that arose from my own knowledge – safety and accurate diagnosis. Using such an economic approach, the cue – 'How can I help this person?' summarises the assessment in terms of a plan of care, the timescale of which can be specified:

- Plan for the first 24 hours
- Give analgesia as prescribed; ask Susan how well it's working
- Susan wants to know what is happening

- Ask Susan to stay on her bed until diagnosis is confirmed (or not)
- Measure her and provide her with anti-embolism stockings
- IV cannula in left hand inserted on admission – monitor anti-coagulant therapy
- Observations as specified on chart

With a more complex situation the BNDU strategy seems to help the nurse identify issues that are relevant to patients, their families and other nurses. Not that this is a unique attribute. Other models that I have used (Roper et al., 1980, Orem 1991 (1992), Roy and Andrews 1991 (1992)) facilitate problem identification that is after all the intention! However, where this particular strategy is different for me is in the sense of the narrative arising from the dialogue.

For example, consider the initial assessment of Ted.

Ted is in his sixties. Recently retired from working as a storesman. He was once a miner. He lives with his wife and has a daughter who lives nearby. He sees her often. He came to the ward two days ago after becoming increasingly ill over the last month. He finds swallowing difficult. He gets breathless easily, but he can still care for himself. We do not know as yet why Ted has these symptoms. He has already been investigated for possible cancer. He says he is most concerned just to know one way or another what is going on. He agrees that his apprehensive; he says that he is taking it 'day by day'. He has lost weight (about half a stone over six weeks). His wife and daughter seem to understand the situation in much the same way as Ted.

This narrative clearly indicated Ted's issues of concern. They were partly due to with psychological issues – uncertainty and fear, and partly to do with physical problems – weight loss and breathlessness. The assessment arose out of several conversations with ideas being checked out with Ted. These conversations enabled me to focus and refocus care on what was most concerning Ted. Conceptual models usually feature an assessment structure and dedicated documentation. Nurses that I have observed and worked with have a tendency to subvert such external structures, finding them restrictive and inhibiting. While the variety and originality that is manifest is invigorating, such a situation is unsatisfactory from the point of view of the need for the collective nursing team to have a consistent approach not least for visiting staff; students, bank and agency staff, and nurses from outside the Unit.

The intention of the assessment strategy being used to elicit a patient's 'situated meaning' (Benner and Wrubel 1987) is explicit (Johns 1991). That the strategy enables this to be articulated is as much to do with the nurses using it, but the process seems to be aided by the use of cues rather than the presentation of a structure into which the nurses try to fit what they have gleaned. With use and adaption the initial pragmatism of an approach which allows for a variety of approaches to recording and presenting information within an identifiable strategy is the potential to unify practice without constraining it.

TELLING A STORY

In the telling of a story from practice, nursing knowledge is preserved in its wholeness, understanding is enhanced (Arnt 1992:287)

Using the BNDU model seems to help the telling of a patient's story, preserving its relevance to them while indicating priorities for the nurse. When collecting my observations, conversations and interpretations, as well as those of others, into a nursing assessment using a more structured approach, the use of headings can prove restrictive. A person's experience does not lend itself to categorisation, especially at the end of a long and busy day (the questionnaire that my colleagues completed suggest that despite their best intentions this is still the time of the day when nursing notes are completed). While, as academic exercises, I have found the use of Orem's self-care deficit model (1991) or Roy's stress adaption theory (Roy and Andrews 1991) useful and illuminating analytical tools, my experience of using them in practice is less fruitful. The notions underlying them are easily diluted by demands on time and thought, even when their concepts are familiar to me. The points concerning the difficulty of complex concepts and language are discussed elsewhere in this chapter.

The example given in the initial assessment of Ted (above) shows how a narrative that is relevant to the patient's situation can arise without the need for an external structure. Writing more or less 'from the hip' was also much quicker than attempting to fit information into prescribed headings. The counter argument that may be posed is that Ted's narrative leaves out a lot information (indeed, for purposes of anonymity it is abbreviated). Here Hall's (1964) point is instructive – 'we can only nurse what the patient allows us to nurse'. After two shifts of spending short periods of time working together, this is what he had shared with me. I had tried to avoid replicating questions that doctors would have already asked him other than checking points from his medical notes that I was unsure about. My intention was to produce a starting point that was relevant, brief, and from where I could plan safe and appropriate care. The reader must take my word that this was indeed the case.

Ted's assessment, for him and for me written here seems hollow in comparison with the scribbled side of A4 paper which I sat and discussed with a very scared but brave man. His words were charged with the emotion of a vital passage of his life and the lives of his family. The bare words contain the pride that was evident when he spoke of his origins in the north of England, the disappointment of becoming ill so soon after retirement, and the resignation to the possibility that he may be gravely ill. His validation of my efforts reassured me that I was directing my energies appropriately. That is not to say my priorities for care were all Ted's, but using the BNDU model seemed to help me find the unity between his agenda and my own and see the inter-relatedness of his problems.

SOME PRACTICAL POINTS

A model for nursing can be perceived as more of a paper exercise than a practical one. My experience of using the BNDU model is that it lends itself to transcending such problems. Using its strategy does not seem to hamper me and it can be applied flexibly to the production of written communications for patients and colleagues. The intention for nursing assessments on 7e is that they should be living documents that can be added to. From the nursing process questionnaires it would also seem that there is a body of opinion that indicates an aspiration amongst the nursing team for members of the multi-disciplinary team to consult nursing notes. A barrier to this is the difficulty of accessing information from nursing notes in their current format. Accordingly, it may be useful for additions to the assessment after the initial narrative account, to be given some sort of heading to indicate what the new information is about, for example – social situation or appetite.[5]

Johns (1991), in describing the model, places most emphasis on the cue questions for assessment. The care planning aspect of nursing process, he suggests, lends itself readily to addressing physical problems. Whilst I would tentatively agree, I would suggest that the formulation of care plans and their content in using the model requires more consideration. The precise function of the care plan is a vexed question.

No single issue, thought, technique, problem or phenomenon has received so much attention, has been as much taught, talked about, worked at, read about and cried over with so little success. No other issue in nursing has caused as much guilt and energy to be misspent. Yet no other piece of paper in a hospital is as devoid of information as that entitled nursing care plan. (Manthey 1980)

A variety of functions are expected from nursing notes; communication, accountability, and auditability, for example. The volume and detail of records required for the above purposes can prove problematic (de la Cuesta 1983, Porter 1991, Howse and Bailey 1992). De la Cuesta's informants saw care plans as 'imposed formalities'. Reed's doctoral work describes how, where the format of nursing documentation is imposed by managers, the relevance of nursing records for nurse themselves is not apparent. Porter, in examining power relations between nurses and doctors, observed that 'the lack of utility value of the nursing process in comparison with the labour required ... has led to disillusionment'. Howse and Bailey noted persistent antipathy towards documentation generally both in review of the literature and in their case study of four Canadian nurses, this antipathy being brought about by inflexible and prescriptive formats as well as lack of confidence and skills in written expression.

There is apparently no clear and unified picture of what nursing records are for. The summary of findings for the Department of Health's investigation (1992) defines the purpose of records vaguely, reporting a need to underpin 'good care' with records. A lack of understanding among nurses of the status of records and their retrospective use as legal evidence is reported. It was also noted that systems of care organisation (primary and team nursing) where patients are better known to nurses resulted in 'less recorded information'. In the same paper the recommendations include the specification of information needed in nursing records in order to use them for workload calculation, as well as the need for service purchasers to specify 'the required standards of nursing records'.

With such uncertainty about the precise function of nursing records it is difficult to plan developments with any accuracy. It is safe to say, however, that extrinsic factors may impinge. For instance, in Oxfordshire the implementation of the Community Care Act has resulted in the hasty introduction of standardised discharge planning package, the explicit reason for the standardised format being ease of audit.

Problems of definition on a large scale do not seem to advance nurses far with the situated question of what nursing records should or should not contain. Johns (1991) suggests care plans should be about physical needs with some form of 'professional notes of their work with patients for use in communication between primary and associate nurses.[6] The nursing team on 7e seem to adapt traditional modes of care planning to varying needs. Where care is self-evident then this fact is recorded on the plan, for example – 'The usual care for someone with a urinary catheter except...'[7]

Where a patient's problem does not lend itself to a concrete goal, then a goal may not be included in the plan, for example where the problem is psycho-social in nature and not easily reduced to the reductionist nature of a care plan. It may be that a particular area of concern is not yet fully understood and that the care plan is used as a focus for gathering information in order to then formulate a plan. This approach was used when it was unclear how much potential a person who had suffered an extensive cerebrovascular accident had for rehabilitation, the goal being to describe the person's behaviour to facilitate assessment.

It may be that an important component of developing practice is to ask similarly pragmatic questions to those contained within the BNDU model: what sort of information do we need to communicate with each other and how do we present it? Experience suggests that the nurse's judgement as to how busy they are and what sort of continuity of care is available to a patient or group of patients to an extent dictates the amount of detail contained in, and the manner of presentation of nursing records.

It may be that a repertoire of methods and approaches is employed which reflects varying needs of patients and changeable pace of work on the ward. Given a consensus amongst the ward team, a regular review process and a means by which new members of the team can be orientated to modes of practice, such an approach could conceivably suffice to ensure a consistent approach from the point of view of communication. Catering for the needs of auditability and accountability is perhaps more problematic since they are essentially outside any single ward's control.

CONSIDERATION OF THE CUE QUESTIONS

The cues are not headings but guides to gather information prompted by the core question 'what information do I need to nurse this person?' My experience of utilising the cues in practice leads me to suggest some adaptations. These adaptations take the form of additional cues and amplifications of the present cues.

WHO IS THIS PERSON?

At times it has proved relevant to include my perception of a patient's 'significant others'. Indeed a holistic standpoint requires that these perspectives are taken into account. Various disease processes as well as the stress of ill-health affect a person's perception of themselves. Whatever the cause, the perceptions of a person's family and friends lend breadth to an understanding of what has happened to a person as a result of ill-health. In an acute medical setting such as 7e where many patients are experiencing multiple pathologies the information provided by those who know the patient can be vital in unravelling what is happening. Presented only with the behaviour of an acutely ill person without this information from others can lead to a distorted perceptions by health practitioners. Two examples come to mind.

1. A man had suffered severe neurological damage. As a result nursing him could present certain practical difficulties if he became uncooperative or even aggressive. Understanding from his family that the way he behaved was an accentuation of how he usually responded to being told what to do to help us to be more patient in our approach to providing him with essential care.

2. A middle-aged man was admitted with signs and behaviour consistent with hyperglycaemia and acute infection. He was confused, irritable, and uncooperative. What was not known was that he also had a psychiatric condition. As he had no immediate family or friends with him at the time of admission it took a matter of days to gather enough information to understand what was happening to him.

This cue guides the practitioner to primarily view the person in their 'wholeness'. Their social cultural world sensitises the practitioner to issues of culture and race and the needs of family and friends – it is much more than simply using family and friends as sources of information about the person.

WHAT HEALTH EVENT BRINGS THIS PERSON INTO HOSPITAL?

Given the holistic basis of the model, it is important to blend together perspectives on the health event underlying a person's contact with health care. A medical diagnosis is just one part of this. From the point of view of a practitioner trying to construct with the patient a picture of their present health event, it is important to find out what they have been experiencing and how they understand it. Such information is necessary for the nursing function of health education and promotion.

The importance of reaching mutual understandings with patients rather than adopting a blanket approach to health education was illustrated when a middle-aged woman was transferred from the Coronary care unit. She had been given both written and verbal information about what had happened, about the effect it would have on her and so on, but it was clear that very little had sunk in. On talking with her about her understanding of her illness she admitted that she knew very little about the workings of the body and did not really understand the explanations given to her. As a result I used diagrams and drawings in an overall approach that avoided giving her too much information at once.[8]

HOW MUST THIS PERSON BE FEELING?

Paying attention to how the person is feeling highlights the dynamic nature of the notion of assessment. A patient's stay in hospital is complex. Their emotional responses are likewise complex and require of the nurse reflexivity and the ability to adapt quickly to a person's changing moods and responses.

HOW HAS THIS EVENT AFFECTED USUAL LIFE PATTERNS AND ROLES?

Consideration of this cue is, as Johns (1991) states, important in setting appropriate goals against a picture of what is normal for a particular person. In essence this is an 'activities of living' question and would lend itself to the adaption of various classifications apart from Roper et al.'s.[9] This cue also has considerable diagnostic power. Increasingly within general hospitals there is an emphasis of expediting discharge or referral of patients as soon as is appropriate. A patient's abilities with regard to activities of living are important in planning for discharge or transfer to other settings (rehabilitation centres, community hospitals, nursing homes, homes with social service support and so on). Within the acute setting it may also be that referral is required to other members of the multi-disciplinary team to provide assistance in some way (physiotherapy, occupational therapy, social work, and so on). In identifying areas of concern, the nurse can also identify the degree of permanence of the changes in life patterns and roles, for instance, how long before someone who has had a heart attack van start driving or to resume a normal sexual relationship.

HOW DOES THE PERSON MAKE ME FEEL?

The intention of this cue shares common ground with the notion of 'bracketing' in phenomenological research (Morse 1991). Phenomenologists describe dealing with their own biases by 'bracketing out' their prejudgments and commitments so as to see new phenomena clearly (Cohen 1987), and with notions of 'emotional competence' in the literature on counselling where practitioners' own concerns do not 'drive or distort' the care that they give (Heron 1990).

The inclusion under the heading of assessment is innovative. Emotional reactions of all kinds may influence the nurse's delivery of care or the equity of care that they deliver to a group of patients. This question epitomises for me the model's utility as a tool to be used in approaching interactions with patients rather than simply as a template for the nursing process. In fact, explicitly recording information about one's feelings about a patient may well be rare in an acute setting. However, considerations of emotional reactions to a patient and their situation will influence communication and so on. Attempting to reflect upon feelings about a patient also provides grounds for comparison with the ideas contained within the ward philosophy.

HOW CAN I HELP THIS PERSON?

The notions underlying this and the following cue lend themselves to that part of the assessment that is diagnostic in nature (Leddy and Pepper 1989). The cue represents a drawing together of information that the nurse has gathered and interpreted. This information is then used to identify strategies for nursing interventions that can be offered to the patient and/or their family.

It may be that for future use with some form of information management system this cue can be linked with a framework of nursing diagnosis. Present taxonomies that are available have been developed in the US. However, given the widespread introduction of computer systems in the UK, it may be wise to consider how approaches to data gathering such as represented by the Burford model can be adapted to allow their use.

WHAT IS IMPORTANT TO MAKE THE PERSON'S STAY IN HOSPITAL COMFORTABLE?

Including a diagnostic cue that is framed from the patient's point of view encourages the nurse to move away from the dilemma posed in previous discussions about nursing process, that of to whose problems is nursing being addressed (de la Cuesta 1983). This and the above cue encourage the nurse to reflect on any discrepancies there might be between their perspective and that of the patient. Thinking about how the patient may be helped is only part of the task, a task completed by exploring what the patient wants. This is far from being a simple task and the components of the debates about the nature of nurse-patient relationships are to be found elsewhere (for example, Gadow (1985), amongst many others).

WHAT SUPPORT DOES THIS PERSON HAVE IN LIFE?

In an acute medical setting where the emphasis is increasingly on swift turnover of patients, the need to address issues concerning the support a patient has in their community is of primary importance. It is therefore a cue that needs to be asked as early as possible after admission; indeed, with the implementation of the 'Care in the Community Act' it is a requirement to screen new admissions to ascertain whether support will be needed after discharge. Separate documentation has been introduced in Oxford in an attempt to standardise the kinds of information gathered about that support available to a patient. For the purposes of learning to employ the Burford model it may be that some areas at least, this cue is better situated higher in the list of cues.[10]

Given the holistic basis of the model, questions of this nature require the nurse to broaden their focus in looking at issues of care after discharge from a variety of points of view. For instance, while a patient's daughter may want to look after a disabled parent at home, it may be necessary to encourage her to explore the needs of her own family as well as her knowledge and skills before final arrangements for discharge are made. This question may benefit from including as sense of what further support is needed.

HOW DOES THE PERSON VIEW THE FUTURE FOR THEMSELVES AND OTHERS?

As Johns (1991) observes, exploration of this question often requires a trusting relationship for patients to expose what their concerns for the future are. Moreover, responses to health crises may be characterised by inaccurate expectations about future problems or abilities. Exploring how the patient and those around them see the future can help set the agenda for the provision of information and referral to other agencies. In the case of Ted above, he anticipated becoming weaker and having more pain, and his wife anticipated not being able to cope looking after him. The measures that we took included making contact with the local hospice services and district nursing and establishing an effective drug regime with Ted learning how some of the drugs worked so that he could tailor them to his needs.

It may be that a useful additional cue my be 'what information does this person need?' In the same way as the cue 'How can I help this person?' and 'what is important to make their stay in hospital comfortable?' have a diagnostic element to them, posing the question 'what information does this person need?' would, along with the addition suggested to the cue 'What further support is needed?' have a similar diagnostic function. These additional cues may facilitate the planning of strategies for health promotion and community support on discharge.[11]

The Burford model's fluid structure seems to lend itself to being an internal tool to make sense of and respond to ever-changing situations.

CLASSIFICATION OF THE CUE QUESTIONS

Using the cue questions to guide my information gathering has led me to loosely classify them as follows:

BASELINE QUESTIONS

- Who is this person?
  - What health event brings this person into hospital?
  - What support does this person have in life?
  - (How does this person make me feel?)

QUESTIONS IDENTIFYING AREAS OF CONCERN

- How must this person be feeling?
  - How has this event affected their usual life pattern and roles? (activities of living)
  - What support does this person have in life?
  - How do they view for themselves and others?
  - (How does this person make me feel?)

DIAGNOSTIC QUESTIONS

- How can I help this person?
  - What is important to make their stay in hospital comfortable?
  - What additional support might they need?
  - What information does this person need?
  - (How does this person make me feel?)

The changing pace and complexity of hospital work, as well as the reflexive approach taken towards individual situations, means that my classification must be flexible. In terms of acute care, I have found that the grouping of the questions helps focus my efforts in a way that reflects the patient's care setting career. An attempt at classification is not so much an attempt to guide the gathering information rather it is an attempt to order it. The question 'how does the person make me feel?' is included in each stage because of its potential for affording perspective on how the nurse is working. It is put in parentheses to denote that thoughts arising from the question are unlikely to be included in permanent records.

CONCLUSIONS

My reflection is of early experiences with using the model and is far from exhaustive. In the first part of this reflection I concluded that there exists a degree of congruence between our mutual visions of practice, and on that basis it was useful to explore using the model in practice. For me, the main power of the model lies in its deceptive simplicity. It is at once pragmatic and profound, useful as an aid to articulating information about a patient and as a framework to guide the building of a relationship between nurse and patient through which both can learn and grow.

NOTES

1 In the 1994 book I had identified these 4 cornerstones of a valid vision. I now integrate the external environment of care within social viability – see Chapter1.

2 The Burford model system for enabling practitioners to realise effective holistic is guided reflection. This is an essential component because this approach enables leaders to live their primary leadership role in guiding practitioners. It enables practitioners to develop reflective skills and becoming reflective practitioners – viewed as an essential aspect of being holistic. It also fosters the learning community and 'living' quality.

3 This approach to leadership shares a similarity with the idea of the holistic leadership approach advocated as necessary within the BNDU model whereby the leader or leadership views itself of service to enable practitioners to take responsibility for their own practice and develop skills necessary to realise effective holistic nursing as a lived reality within a community of inquiry (see Chapter 1).

4 It is helpful to point out that a philosophy or vision for practice is always evolving in light of new ideas, new knowledge and experience. However, it must be a 'complete' statement to give direction and meaning to practice. In light of knowing 'social viability' 7e may return to their philosophy and consider whether it should reflect 'social viability'.

5 Note the use of Special Intervention sheets for drawing attention to particular issues of care pulled out from the general narrative.

6 Care plans as part of the nursing process were discontinued in favour of narrative simply because review of care plans indicated they had no real value. Clearly narratives included a plan of care supplemented by special Intervention sheets (see Chapter 4).

7 At Burford we developed a series of protocols incorporated within specific standards of care to guide 'routine' aspects of care, for example mouth care, catheter care. Hence the notes could state – care as protocol except... (see Chapter 7).

8 Garbett's focus on health education is not the focus of this cue – this might be expected under a later cue – how can I help this person? However Garbett's inclusion of this experience under this cue illustrates the difficulty practitioners unused to the BNDU cues may 'know' where to place certain information especially when they have been socialised into filling in headings or boxes.

9 As I noted in response to Sutherland's account (Chapter 8) – practitioners will necessarily gravitate to learnt ways of assessment even with the application of the Burford model. Yet structuring this cue (or indeed any other) defeats the holistic object – persons are not simply 'activities of living'. Such thinking becomes redundant with using the cues. Any setting adopting the Burford model will naturally give practitioners support to use the model appropriately but never losing sight of its holistic intent.

10 Given the significance of the cue 'what support does this person have in life?' Garbett feels it could be listed higher in the sequence of cues. However, this misses the point that the cues are always at work from admission to discharge through a continuous process of assessment, action and evaluation. Hence in settings where discharge issues are urgent such as acute medical setting with the persistent problem of bed blocking, the practitioners will give this cue the attention it requires.

11 Garbett proposes additional questions – 'what information does this person need?' and 'what further support is needed?' Practitioners adopting the BNDU model will inevitably adapt it to suit their own visions and practicalities. I do not consider these additional necessary from the perspective of practice at Burford. It is like adding braces to the belt –however this begins to resemble a more concrete and ultimately a less flexible model, reflecting the influence of his experience with previous models with the risk of fitting the person into the classification rather than using the cues creatively to gather information.

REFERENCES

Arnt M J (1992) Caring as everydayness. *Journal of Holistic Nursing* 10(4); 285–293.

Bagust A, Slack R, and Oakley J (1992) *Ward nursing quality and grade mix.* York Health Economics Consortium, University of York, York.

Benner P and Wrubel J (1987) *The primacy of caring.* Addison–Wesley, Menlo Park.

Benner P and Wrubel J (1989) *The primacy of caring: stress and coping in health and illness.* Addison–Wesley, Menlo Park.

Chapman P (1990) A critical perspective. In *Models for nursing 2* (Eds. B Kershaw and J Salvage) Scutari Press, Harrow.

Cohen M S (1987) An historical overview of the phenomenological movement. image. *Journal of Nursing Scholarship* 19(1); 31–34.

De la Cuesta C (1983) The nursing process from development to implementation. *Journal of Advanced Nursing* 8; 365–371.

Department of Health (1992) *Summary of report of nursing records study: good practice.* (PL/CNO 92) HMSO, London.

Draper P (1990) The development of theory in British nursing: current position and future prospects. *Journal of Advanced Nursing* 15(1); 12–15.

Gadow S (1985) Nurse and patient: the caring relationship. In *Caring, curing, coping* (Eds. A H Bishop and J R Scudder) University of Alabama Press, Birmingham.

Gordon D (1984) Research application: identifying the use and misuse of formal models in nursing practice. In *From novice to expect' excellence and power in nursing* (Ed. P Benner) Addison-Wesley, Menlo Park.

Gruending (1985) Nursing theory: a vehicle for professionalization? *Journal of Advanced Nursing* 10(6); 553–558.

Hall L (1964) Nursing– what is it? *Canadian Nurse* 60(2); 150–4.

Hancock C (1992) Nurses and skill mix: what are the issues? *Paper presented at the Nurses skill mix conference* St Bartholomews Hospital, London.

Helt E and Jellinek R C (1988) In the wake of cost cutting, nursing productivity and quality improve. *Nursing Management* 19(6); 36–48.

Heron J (1990) *Helping the client.* Sage, London.

Howse E and Bailey J (1992) Resistance to documentation – nursing research issue. *International Journal of Nursing Studies* 29(4); 371–380.

Johns C (1989) Developing a philosophy for practice part 1. *Nursing Practice* 3(1); 2–5.

Johns C (1991) The Burford Nursing Development Unit holistic model of nursing practice. *Journal of Advanced Nursing* 16; 1090–1098.

Johns C (1992) Ownership and harmonious team: barriers to developing the therapeutic team in primary nursing. *Journal of Clinical Nursing* 1; 89–94.

Johnson D E (1974) Development of theory: a requisite fornursing as a primary health profession. *Nursing Research* 23(5); 373–377.

Leddy S and Pepper J (1989) *Conceptual basis for professional nursing* (second edition) J B Lippincott, Philadelphia.

Lister P (1987) The misunderstood model. *Nursing Times* 83(41); 40–42.

Manthey M (1980) *The practice of primary nursing.* Blackwell scientific Publications, Oxford.

May C (1992) Nursing work, nurses' knowledge, and the subjectification of the patient. *Sociology of Health and Illness* 14(4); 472–487.

Miller A (1985) The relationship between nursing theory and nursing practice. *Journal of Advanced Nursing* 10(5); 417–424.

Morse J (1991) *Qualitative nursing research: a contemporary dialogue*. Sage, Newbury Park.

Orem D E (1991) *Nursing concepts of practice* (fourth edition) C V Mosby, St. Louis.

Pembrey S (1984) Nursing care: nursing progress. *Journal of Advanced Nursing* 9(6); 539–47.

Porter S (1991) A participant observation study of power relations between nurses and doctors in a general hospital. *Journal of Advanced Nursing* 16; 728–735.

Roper N, Logan W W, and Tierney A (1980) *The elements of nursing*. Churchill Livingstone, Edinburgh.

Roy C and Andrews H A (1991) The Roy adaption model; the definitive statement. In *Conceptual models for nursing practice* (Ed. J P Sisca) Appleton and Lange, California.

Ryan D (1989) *Project 1999 – the support hierarchy as the management contribution to project 2000*. Discussion paper, Department of Nursing Studies, University of Edinburgh, Edinburgh.

Waterworth K and Luker K (1990) Reluctant collaborators; do patients want to be involved in decisions concerning care? *Journal of Advanced Nursing* 15;971–976.

Wright S (1989) *Changing nursing practice*. Edward Arnold, London.

CHAPTER 14

Peter and Sam[1]

Christopher Johns

PREFACE

The narrative 'Peter and Sam' is my personal exemplar of being a holistic practitioner. The experience took place at a hospice that had implemented the Burford NDU model[2] where I practiced one day a week as a holistic therapist.[3]

PETER AND SAM

It is mid-February. Another cold morning driving to the hospice along dark slippery lanes. I'm late, but a whisper tells me be patient, not to rush into the darkness where danger lurks for the careless.

At the hospice, I am asked if I can do anything for the odour in Peter's room. I do not know him. I am told he is close to death. Just 52 years old. As an aromatherapist I am often asked to combat unpleasant odour – what is euphemistically referred to as perfuming. Christine[4] [a staff nurse] pulls me aside 'Could you also offer Sam, Peter's wife, something? She's very distressed.' I tend not to read the patient's narrative preferring to find the person to tell their story. Later when writing my notes I could read the patient's narrative as necessary.[5]

Peter's room opens onto a corridor shared by several single rooms. Walking down the corridor, I observe the woman who sits outside Peter's room. People are gathered around her. She looks up and gazes at me as I slowly approach. I know it is Sam even though we have not met before.

I gently inquire 'Sam?'

She nods. Her distress is palpable, rippling through her even as she endeavours to contain it. I inform her who I am and inquire 'have you been here all night?'

Again she nods.
I say 'You must be tired?'
She replies 'Yes... I am but it's OK.... [silence].... I need to be here.'
I say 'I know.'
I know because I can read the signs. I have heard this story many times before. It is legend.

Holistic Practice in Healthcare: The Burford NDU Person-centred Model, Second Edition. Edited by Christopher Johns.

We move into Peter's room and gaze at him. He looks peaceful, his breathing slightly noisy. She holds one hand and I take the other. He is not responsive even though yesterday Sam says he had a jacuzzi bath. Today is another story. An unfolding drama.

Holding his hand I begin to tune into him, feeling for his wavelength to connect with him and tell him through my touch that I care for him. No words spoken. We dwell in the silence that lies thick between us. Meeting a family for the first time under these conditions is never easy. The air is thick with emotional tension. Uncertain as how best to respond I buy myself time by continuing to hold Peter's hand and sit silently with him, *listening* to him, being mindful of what is happening about me and within me, bringing myself into the right space to give therapy. And yet I feel pressure from both myself and from Sam to act quickly, to grasp at a solution to ease Peter's suffering in the face of the other's and my own anxiety. I am mindful of not falling into a fix-it mentality. Being mindful is being patient, mindful of not rushing into the darkness, of being careless.

I am mindful of the nurses' request to combat the odour. It isn't pleasant. I imagine it oozing from the rotting cavities. To sit by your dying husband waiting for his death is not easy. To sit with the smell of his rotting body must exacerbate the suffering.

I do not mention the odour to Sam. I wonder if she has acclimatised herself to it. I suggest to Sam that therapeutic touch might help Peter?

She says 'Anything that might help please try.'

Seeing her so vulnerable, so desperate I want to hold her and say it's OK. She gives a thin smile as if she knows and seeks to reassure me. She doesn't ask what therapeutic touch involves and I do not inform her. She is absorbed in his and her own suffering.

I place my hand above Peter's chest and abdomen and sense the heat and pressure of the cancer.

Sam, intrigued, asks 'What are you doing?'

I say 'I intend by moving my hands across Peter's body it will help reduce the heat and pressure from his body and ease his suffering.'

Saying *ease his suffering* seems to reassure Sam. The word suffering is so evocative, confrontational even, as if it dares to name the palpable tension.

I might have added – 'and ease your suffering as well'. I don't say this because I know it would be a distraction – that she would say she didn't want any attention for herself.

I know that to treat Peter is to treat Sam especially as she continues to hold his hand.

I centre myself, mindful of my presence as *lifting energy*.[6] And for 20 minutes or so we dwell in silence as I practice.

Afterwards Sam says 'Peter seems so much more peaceful and his breathing is easier.'

The room is very still and I sense that she too, is now easier.

I had intended the therapeutic touch would combat the odour, and indeed it has diminished. I know this from experience as if the odour emanates from a restless spirit.[7]

Sam informs me that she has been at the hospice at his bedside since Peter's admission. She knows he is dying and waits anxiously. Waiting is a constant theme through my reflections. As a therapist I journey alongside people so they are not alone but mindful not to be intrusive in the waiting. However, Sam seems to welcome my company. She says 'It's only a week since his diagnosis. For eight months he was treated for stomach reflux whist the cancer ate away his pancreas. He experienced great pain, had lost 5 stone in weight, then the jaundice appeared and now this....'

Her words trail off as her tears move close to the surface.

Such history is not uncommon. Questions that require answers but now is not the time.

Her contained anger alongside the despair of his dying fuelling the deep conflict she feels. But now she must give her attention to Peter. Sam suffers not just Peter's dying but the anguish of his misdiagnosis. Peter is a young man; his life ripped away.

I try and empathise with Sam but struggle to connect with the turmoil I sense inside her, inside the container. How do I begin to understand her thoughts and feelings?

I ask 'how are you feeling'?

No words. Perhaps no words are needed to feel her despair as she sits by Peter. Perhaps my inquiry was futile, banal... finding the right words to say is sometimes difficult. Sam follows me outside his room and says 'I am bursting inside... it is our wedding anniversary today... I couldn't sleep last night... I kept dreaming I was at home and reaching for him in the empty bed.'

She bursts open. Her tears cascade like a burn in full spring flow. She is tossed on a raging sea of grief. I feel as if I pick my way through the bobbing debris, the desolation that cancer leaves in its wake.

'Is there something I can offer you... to help you relax?'

I feel the unspoken demand to care for this life put into my hands.[8]

Sam is silent and then as if she has been thinking deeply she says 'That's kind of you.... I've slept at times... I'm really tried, exhausted... struggling being with Peter... but no. I don't want any treatment. I want you to give attention to Peter.'

Her look is plaintiff. Sam wants no distraction from her bedside quest. Like many spouses she feels that any attention for her would be taking attention away from Peter. However, I have already eased her suffering with the Therapeutic Touch.

I offer to set up an aroma-stone to make the room smell more pleasant and induce a sense of calm. She accepts my offer but does not want a strong heady smell. I find myself deliberating which oils to use. I do not give Sam choice but chose bergamot. She likes its smell. Bergamot is well known to combat anxiety.[9] I am cognisant of Worwood's words[10]

> *We may cry inside, our hearts aching, but bergamot will lighten the heart and dispel self-criticism and blame.*

Perfect words for the occasion. Sometimes I read these spiritual descriptors to those sitting at the bedside but not this time, even though I carry Worwood's book in my satchel. I sense the words would be inappropriate to say despite their appropriateness to the moment. I move away leaving Sam at the bedside holding Peter's hand.

Later, I attend the shift report and give an account of my work with Peter and Sam this morning. I share my views on combating odour. I assert that it's too easy to assume the odour has a physical cause, that perhaps it is a manifestation of despair? Someone says the room definitely smells better. Successful perfuming.

Christine chips in 'Did you give Sam a treatment?'

I reply 'Not directly, only through giving Peter Therapeutic Touch... she held his hand... she didn't want any attention from him.'

I tell them about Sam's wedding anniversary and her despair emphasising my presence of being with her and Peter and the significance of lifting energy. No comment. The shift report moves on. There is no dialogue, simply the giving of information. I sense the way their partial listening has filtered out information that does not fit their agenda.

A ripple of despondency ripples over me. I sense my frustration hit the wall and ripple backwards yet no-one seems to notice. I sense my poise on edge. And yet I keep quiet rather than voice the contradiction I feel with holistic practice and the inadequate nature of the communication between us. The illusion of the collaborative team exposed. I do not try to shift it, at least not now. I know I work in the margins. I know I am in the right place to work as a holistic practitioner yet not really part of the collective team. Yet by attending the shift report I make my presence felt, imposing myself into the team, moving in from the margins. The nurses are not used to a complementary therapist imposing a view, reflected in the small space on the complementary therapy sheet allocated to 'comment' where I am expected to write [reflect?] on my interventions. I am aware that other complementary therapists simply write – 'relaxed' – as if the therapist role is simply that – to aid relaxation. However, as is my custom, I write an account of my experience with Peter and Sam in both the complementary therapist sheet and in the patient notes. I do this deliberately to confront the 'normal' procedure that I find unsatisfactory and marginalising.

Imagine if I 'invaded' the multi-professional meeting and talked about 'the spiritual' how the chaplain would feel elbowed; or if I wrote about despair the psychologist would take offence; or about physical pain the doctors would curtly rebuke me; or that if I gave advice on constipation or helped someone get to the toilet I would be reprimanded by nurses for exceeding my role. The patient and holistic practitioner both fragmented within professional territorial. Writing this narrative prompts me to inform and remind those reading the notes of holistic practice, notably that easing suffering is the acknowledged intent of palliative care, not just for the person dying but also for the family.

Before leaving the hospice I return to the room to say goodbye to Peter and Sam to wish them well on their difficult journey. Sam remains by the bedside maintaining her death vigil. I can imagine the knots tightening in her neck and along her shoulders. Being a massage therapist shapes my gaze!

Like a stranger I appear and then disappear from their torn lives. It is an extraordinary privilege to dwell with people so intensely, so intimately, just for a short time. And for a brief moment I imagine Avalokitishvara, the Bodhisattva of compassion, wrapping us in his arms of compassion. I am left with a good feeling despite their suffering. I did not meet Peter or Sam again. I learnt that he died two days later.

COMMENTARY

Such is my practice, entering the hospice and finding myself in the midst of such drama. Writing this narrative raises many issues for me as I aspire to realise holistic practice, developing insights to inform my future practice. As always, I wonder if I could have been more available to Peter and Sam in the brief moment we dwelt together. I wonder how other practitioners respond to them? I sensed Christine's concern when she asked 'could you also offer Sam, Peter's wife, something. She's very distressed.' How we care for her is vital to ease her suffering now and after Peter's death – so when she looks back she will feel the presence of people who helped ease Peter's suffering, and with it her own. That people were there for her.

My response to Sam and Peter was as I found it. It would have been impossible to plan such care. It illustrates how much of holistic practice is intuitive and creative, in response to shifting patterns. Holistic practice is always being open to what is unfolding, moving through chaos held together by the intent to realise holistic practice.[11] It is opening possibility for caring and healing through diverse therapies and generally being mindful of creating an environment that facilitates the person's growth and healing.[12]

As a holistic therapist (in contrast to my role as a nurse) I claimed autonomy to organise my practice and deliver therapy as I felt appropriate in collaboration with my peers, nurses and other disciplines. I am not there to 'fix' problems at the dictate of nurses redolent of a symptomatic treatment approach.

My approach is how I perceive the primary nurse role. The hospice had chosen not to implement primary nursing feeling that it would be too divisive. Instead they decided to continue their normal practice of allocating nurses to patients on a daily basis. As such, I felt relationships (as with Peter and Sam) were fragmented. The nursing notes had not reflected Sam's distress even though they had adopted the reflexive narrative approach. It reminded me how new technology can be accommodated into normal practice. Perhaps my writing in the notes will remind others of holistic practice.

My rather cynical reference to other disciplines reflects how practice can be fragmented through these different specialists each with their finger in the pie claiming authority for this part or that part of Peter. These specialists did not routinely attend the office bound handover. Yet I feel as a holistic practitioner responding to the whole persons (Peter and Sam) I step over disciplinary boundaries as appropriate yet mindful of 'being out of my depth' when I can confer with others if Sam and Peter wanted that.

I find myself constantly (both deliberately and inadvertently) undermining the 'old' hospice culture to create an environment whereby holistic care can be realised. In doing so, I become political but careful not to become marginalised, especially with nurses who 'control' the workplace. As the saying goes 'Rome wasn't built in a day' – yet it is difficult being a lone ranger without my 'Burford' authority to lead and drive holistic practice. Yet I can make a difference. I decide to attend handovers and multi-disciplinary meetings more regularly to assert my presence and perspective and remind the 'team' that the primary ethos of palliative care is to ease suffering (as indicated in the WHO definition of palliative care) more than symptomatic treatment. Then practitioners might first see 'the person' rather than the symptoms they present.

NOTES

1 A version of this narrative was published in *Becoming a Reflective Practitioner*, third edition (2009:24–28).

2 The hospice considered it already practiced holistic care although this was not espoused in their written vision for practice at this time. However, the culture of the hospice was medically dominated with a primary focus on symptomatic care. It was on the hospice agenda to revise the vision taking a bottom-up approach rather than an organisational approach. However, it had implemented the Burford NDU assessment strategy and narrative as a way of recording and communicating the patient's story.

3 Working at the hospice enabled me to maintain my clinical credibility to teach end-of-life care at the University besides the satisfaction and fulfilment of being a holistic practitioner. I use narratives in my teaching as the basis to stimulate dialogue around significant aspects of end-of-life care practice and to trigger students' own reflections and to contextualise theory so its value to inform practice is immediately appreciated. The notion of clinical credibility is vital – how can a teacher 'teach' holistic practice unless they practice and reflect on it? If not, then teachers can only teach it theoretically (if taught at all). This is called 'running in place' (as noted in the Preface). Being clinically present also enabled me to guide students on clinical placement, role-modelling holistic practice.

4 Christine was Peter's allocated nurse for the shift. Primary nursing as a system for delivering holistic practice was resisted due to its perceived threat to disrupt normal patterns of organising care through daily

patient allocation. However, it is not imperative practice settings adopt primary nursing. As I highlight in Chapter 5, primary nursing may be best suited for delivering holistic practice because it most facilitates the practitioner-person relationship and the development of responsibility.

5 If I was Peter's allocated practitioner I would have read the notes after speaking with Peter (as able) in order to evaluate Peter's care as planned to continue it as appropriate. I cannot emphasise enough the significance of speaking with Peter (and in this case Sam) before evaluating the planned care – this is the benefit of walkabout handovers – see Chapter 4.

6 *Lifting energy* – see Chapter 1.

7 Johns C (2004). *Being Mindful, Easing Suffering: Reflections on Palliative Care.* Jessica Kingsley Publishing, London.

8 Logstrup K E (1997). The ethical demand. University of Notre Dame Press, Notre Dame, IN.

9 Davis P (1999) *Aromatherapy A-Z.* C W Daniel, Saffron Walden.

10 Worwood V (1999 *The fragrant heavens.* Doubleday, London).

11 From a chaos theory perspective, the intent to realise holistic practice is the strange attractor around which practice patterns itself. Hence, whilst my experience with Peter and Sam may appear random to the observer, it has an inherent order.

12 The expanse of a holistic healing environment is extensively addressed in Helming B and Shields D (2020) (Eds.) Dossey and Keegan's Holistic Nursing: a handbook for practice (eighth edition) Jones and Bartlett, Burlington.

Holistic Practice Matters

CHAPTER 15

Christopher Johns

Holistic practice matters. It matters to me as a nurse and it matters to me as a person needing health care. Just this past week (November 2022) I was admitted to hospital with acute appendicitis. Everywhere around the hospital I noticed stickers reminding practitioners of dignity as if dignity was a problem to be remedied. Yet, few nurses introduced themselves to me or addressed me by my name. Without names there is no human connection. I felt like an object. The morning after my operation a charge nurse arrived at the bedside on the 'drug round'. Without saying a word he wrote my name up on the board and then his name 'Paul' as named nurse and 'Stacey', the name of a Health care assistant. I asked him 'Are you Paul?' He said 'Yes' and apologised. That was the extent of our talk. He went to the next patient and said 'Hello, I'm Paul' as if he had been reminded about dignity. He did not ask how I was feeling or inquire about my low blood pressure all night and scanty urine output. He didn't inquire about my pain or ask to see the wound or talk about discharge probably later that day. He didn't inquire if I had any concerns. There was simply no connection.

Shortly afterwards, I was approached by a Health Care assistant intent on taking my blood pressure. Like Paul, she didn't introduce herself and did not address me by my name. I asked 'Are you Stacey?' She said yes as if it didn't matter. She was there to do a task not to develop a relationship. I was just a task to do. Run of the mill stuff on a surgical ward. I sensed that the named nurse routine was purely a formality that had no meaning. Observing Paul during the morning he was very functional, tying up the laundry bags. He didn't inquire if I needed help in the bathroom. I asked myself 'Do I expect too much?' 'Does it matter if nurses like Paul make no connection?' Of course it matters. Human connection is lifting for the person. The stickers reminding practitioners of dignity acknowledges that fact, that people have names, have identities, have feelings and suffer from illness that brings them into hospital. My experience was a sobering reminder that holistic practice is not a reality on this ward and yet it only required a caring attitude to make the connection, to feel human rather than an object being processed (and not very competently) through the health-fixing machine. As I left the ward to be shunted into the discharge lounge to make space for the next person, Paul was not about. No information about wound care or pain management of follow-up. It was a demoralising experience, not just for myself, but for nursing in general. And yet, it only needed a turn of the mind to view his practice holistically. Holism is primarily an attitude. Then he might look at me, introduce himself and ask himself 'who is this person?' It doesn't matter if I am going home that day. A holistic attitude naturally asks such questions as set out in the Burford assessment strategy. Maybe it will take him a little longer but

Holistic Practice in Healthcare: The Burford NDU Person-centred Model, Second Edition. Edited by Christopher Johns.

then the care assistant can tie up the laundry bags. And then perhaps to infect his staff with a similar attitude through dialogue – 'what do we aspire to in our collective practice?' Or put another way 'what matters to us as nurses?'

Realising holistic practice is a matter of urgency when set against a background of continuous reports of poor health and social care. Holistic practice matters to so many practitioners who lead contradictory and unsatisfactory lives because they are unable to deliver holistic practice resulting in low moral, burnout and poor practice. No wonder that the most caring practitioners leave.

If holistic practice matters then practitioners need practice environments and development to enable it to be realised. They need committed and skilled holistic teachers and leaders. The Burford NDU is such an environment as evidenced through the practitioner's narratives that illuminate the impact holistic practice makes for persons and their families and for themselves.

Realising holistic practice will be a significant culture shift for many readers. It is not easy to accomplish as an individual practitioner. It requires collective action and leadership to drive the necessary culture shift (shock). The two biggest challenges (threats?) to realising holistic practice are firstly, the transactional organisation that characterises healthcare organisations anxiously concerned with outcomes, targets, fiscal security and their own smooth running to the extent that they have lost sight of the primary purpose to treat and care for persons, both staff and patients, despite hoisting 'people investor' banners. It is worth noting that the Burford NDU model was created at Burford hospital without extra resource. It worked because practitioners wanted it, were committed to it, was supported by the organisation, and went the extra mile for it. The practitioners felt liberated to practice creatively in tune with their collective holistic beliefs.

Secondly, to re-vision the nursing curriculum that manifestly does not prepare practitioners to become holistic practitioners. It requires University nursing and healthcare curriculum to implement a holistic and reflective curriculum (Johns 2022)[1] around core holistic values to prepare students for holistic practice reinforced by mentors in practice – thus demanding that students are placed in acknowledged holistic practice settings. Fundamentally holistic practice cannot be taught; it can only be learnt by creating space for students to explore and learn through their experiences informed by extant theory and ideas as relevant.

However, I know from personal experience that Universities are stuck in a traditional rut because teachers resist change for many reasons (Johns 2022). It requires political and professional bodies such as the Nursing, Midwifery Council and Royal College of Nursing in the UK to exert their influence. It requires every Chief nurse sitting on healthcare boards and every matron strolling about to become holistic leaders to champion holistic practice. The significance of holistic leadership cannot be overstated.[2]

Writing this, I feel a bit like Gordon Ramsey and his USA kitchen nightmare scenarios attempting to shake up and reform what has become moribund and unsatisfactory poor service. Unfortunately most patients do not have choice – the NHS is what it is and people have to put up with it rather like a care lottery, some saying that care was good but many others complaining bitterly.

THE BURFORD NDU CONCEPTUAL MODEL

Drawing together the threads of the Burford NDU model explicated through the book I have constructed a conceptual map (Table 15.1) to illustrate how the five organisational systems integrate into the whole picture. This map has been adapted from the Julia Farr Centre NDU

Table 15.1 The Burford NDU model conceptual map

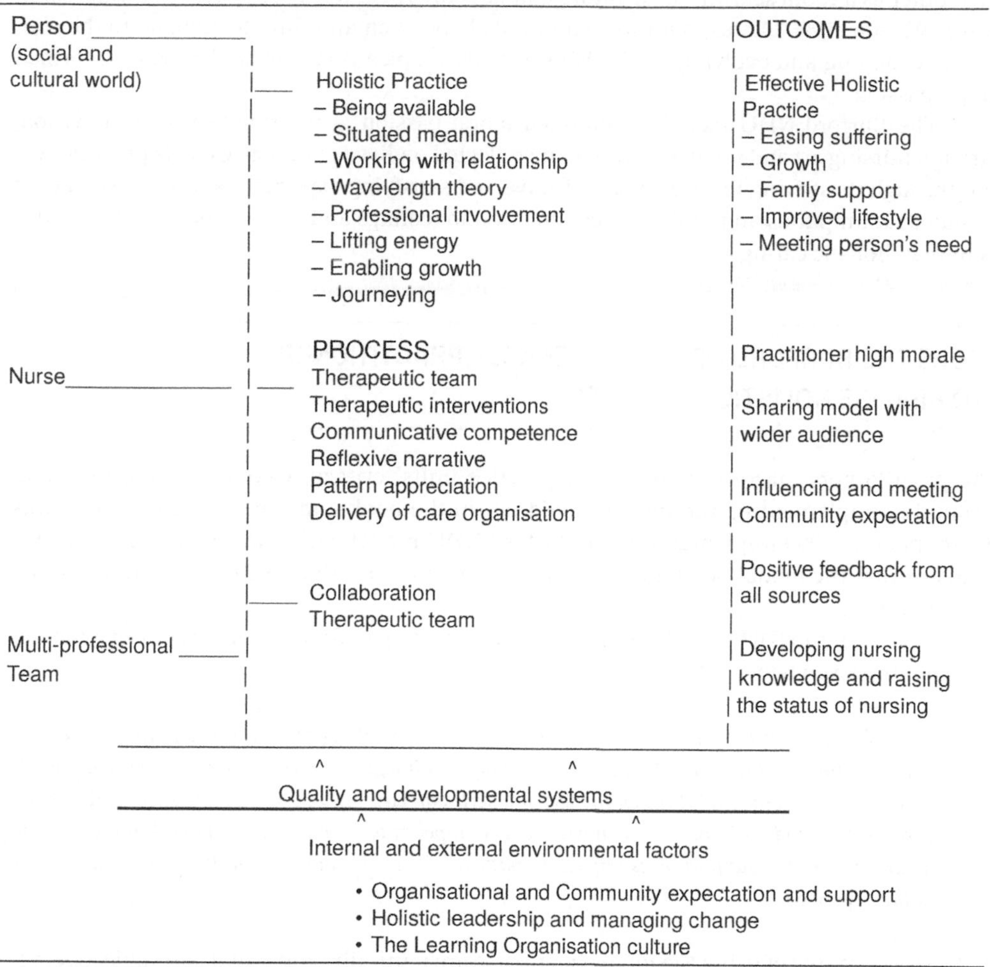

VISION

Elements	Process	Outcomes
Person (social and cultural world)	Holistic Practice – Being available – Situated meaning – Working with relationship – Wavelength theory – Professional involvement – Lifting energy – Enabling growth – Journeying	OUTCOMES Effective Holistic Practice – Easing suffering – Growth – Family support – Improved lifestyle – Meeting person's need
Nurse	PROCESS Therapeutic team Therapeutic interventions Communicative competence Reflexive narrative Pattern appreciation Delivery of care organisation	Practitioner high morale Sharing model with wider audience Influencing and meeting Community expectation Positive feedback from all sources
Multi-professional Team	Collaboration Therapeutic team	Developing nursing knowledge and raising the status of nursing

^ ^

Quality and developmental systems

^ ^

Internal and external environmental factors

- Organisational and Community expectation and support
- Holistic leadership and managing change
- The Learning Organisation culture

map (O'Brien and Pope 1994) itself adapted from the revised Burford NDU conceptual map (Johns 1991, 1994) illustrating how dialogue between Unit settings reflexively informs and develops ideas.

As O'Brien and Pope (1994:187–8) wrote

> *The conceptual framework that initially evolved from the reflective interpretation of NDU nurses' experience at Julia Farr Centre has come to be challenged through an evolving dialogue, established between Christopher Johns and the authors of this chapter. The commitment to reflective practice has encouraged nurses to interpret and articulate their own evolving practice rather than slavishly adopting the dictates of a particular nursing model. Arising out of this discourse came the decision 'to construct a tailor made model of nursing from the practitioners' own values and beliefs' (citing Johns 1991:1091).*

Constructing a conceptual map can be likened to a 'common room' in the way it sets out the Burford NDU model concepts as a room sets out its furniture and how the concepts relate to each other as a room sets out its furniture and how the room itself is set within a wider landscape. Watson (1990) states that this room needs to be open and fluid to respond to the constantly changing and evolving world. Watson makes a plea that this landscape is 'informed moral passion'.

The Burford NDU model is 'informed moral passion' – informed through its vision, through nursing art and science, through the reflected on lived experiences of its practitioners and through its striving for ever more effective and satisfying experiences. It is passionate in its stated assumptions and in its explicit attention to feelings and in its pursuance of practice as human holistic caring.

DOES THE BURFORD NDU MODEL ENABLE PRACTITIONERS TO REALISE HOLISTIC PRACTICE?

The practitioners' narratives and other practice units' critical accounts considering and evaluating implementing the model as laid out in the book and other published accounts (Graham et al. 1999 implementing the Burford NDU model within a surgical setting), give evidence that the model facilitates realising holistic practice that makes a difference to the care of persons.

The Burford NDU model was singled out as lacking definition, modes of implementation and unproven benefit (MacKintosh 1998). She states –

> *These failings can be found in much of the literature describing the Buford reflection in nursing model (Johns 1998a, 1998b, 1998c) which attempts to integrate reflective practice into a clinically grounded nursing model through the use of a series of 'cues'. Much of the published evidence, regarding the model's impact on clinical practice appears to be based on personal anecdote, and again, evidence in support of its impact on patient care is of a mainly qualitative and descriptive nature. (p. 556)*

Reflective accounts of using the model in practice are naturally contextual and subjective, yet written from a reflective perspective whereby practitioners are able to stand back and view experience more objectively mindful of their partial perspectives. The accounts within the original Burford NDU nook (1994) were not cited by Mackintosh. Indeed Mackintosh reviews the literature from her own partial eye, seeing and interpreting what she wants to read to support her prejudice against reflective evidence. As Wilber (1998) notes, different ways of knowing are paradigmatic with their own specific rules of injunction as to what counts as truth (see Table 15.2). Reflective accounts are located in the subjective individual quadrant (top left) and who better to know their own truth than practitioners who have been schooled to be critically reflective, so whilst subjective and contextual, their subjectivity is critically moderated through guided reflection. The collective accounts are located in the subjective collective (bottom left). Hence different paradigms have competing notions of the nature of 'truth'. To dispute subjective truth then every survey, interview, and psychometric test is flawed, tainted with the 'suspicion of authenticity' and perhaps more so because the truth is obscured behind an objective illusion.

Table 15.2 Paradigmatic ways of knowing

	Interior Left-hand paths Subjective	Exterior Right-hand paths Objective
Individual	'I' personal fit (authenticity) Truth injunction: truthfulness	'IT' behavioural fit (what is observed fits the facts) Truth injunction: propositional truth statistic
Collective	'WE' cultural fit (mutual understanding) Truth injunction: justness Intersubjective	'IT' functional fit (how things fit within the whole) Truth injunction: statistic Interobjective

HELEN'S ACCOUNT[3]

Consider Helen's account of using the Burford NDU model. How compelling is it as 'evidence' to support the efficacy of the Burford NDU model to enable practitioners to realise effective holistic practice.

Helen is a nutrition clinical nurse specialist working within a general hospital. She was inspired to implement the Burford NDU model into her practice and requested I offered her guided reflection to help her realise her holistic vision.

Helen: 'Using the Burford NDU model confronted me with the fact that people have real feelings. It has provoked a chain of thinking – "why do I go to visit these patients?" "What am I trying to achieve?" I got an unpleasant feeling of not offering them anything except maybe to increase their safety. I am actively making this effort to see them as people, to see them differently from how I have been seeing them.'

CJ: 'Does this lead to increased satisfaction?'

Helen: 'Yes! Although it makes it tougher. It has challenged my "task" approach. Now I probably see fewer patients in a day. That is itself frustrating but I am more satisfied with what I do.'

CJ: 'A key aspect of your work is managing time and priorities?'

Helen: 'It's the crux of the CNS role. I don't want to "police" others' work but that's what has happened! At least the danger of it, if that hasn't totally happened. It may also be a problem of being part-time. I don't work enough hours, or maybe it's a problem about the way I work, the "beast the clock" thing. The reflective cues "How is this person feeling?" and "How do I feel about this person?" keep popping in my head. I had situation with a patient, Kim; it changed the whole way the experience went. She is 26 with Crohn's disease. She has a nasty fistula pouring fluid. She is on total parental nutrition (TPN). I visited her on the ward. Her dressing had been done. The "Hickman line" should have been fixed in. She had sat on it and pulled it out. The doctor said he would sort another one but she had said "No". I went in. I knew she would not get better without a new line. My intention was to be forceful just like the doctors. And then I stopped myself. I asked myself "why am I acting like this?" I noted my feelings – that I was anxious that she was not safe without the TPN. I asked her how she was feeling. She was reacting against having TPN forced on her. She has been like this for two years now. Her life has been turned upside down with no feeling of control – her only control was to say "No". I confronted her with this – "Is this how you have been feeling?" She said "Yes, that's exactly how I am feeling. I'm not having it!" I sat and talked it through with her. In the end we negotiated a compromise – that she could go home for the weekend to spend it with her children without the line and return on Monday to have the line re-sited. We agreed.'

CJ: 'You saw the person instead of the problem?'

Helen: 'It was wonderful. I went home beaming! Since then I have had other situations with doctors rushing her. For example, her Hb was 6.7 and she needed a blood transfusion. She told them to 'push off' saying "I'm a honorary Jehovah's Witness." But give her time and she will mull it over. Eventually she said she was happy with this. When they put the second line in the intention was to give her two units of blood through it before the TPN. I said to the consultant on the ward round "No, that line is for the TPN." I confronted him. He agreed with me. But two to three weeks later the doctors tried to give her another transfusion through the "Cuff Cath". She said to them "No your not. Helen said No!" The doctor went to the consultant who again agreed with me that they were not doing that. I had told Kim why it was important, that it contaminated the line with the risk of CVP sepsis.'

COMMENTARY

Helen's account is her confessional wakeup call that patients are people, illustrating the perverse influence of the medical model. The power of just two of the Burford NDU model cues to jolt her out of her routine complacency prompting the question 'what am I trying to achieve?' and shifting from a task approach to a holistic approach.

Helen knew her therapeutic response was to be available to Kim, to tune into Kim's wave length and understand the meanings and feelings Kim gave to her illness to give Kim control over her life. Kim needed to reclaim her own body that had been taken away from her by the medical system intent on fixing it but not paying attention to who she was – the classic mind-body split. In repositioning herself Helen became a space in which Kim could reflect her feelings and reclaim her body. Helen's role was no longer to fix Kim's body but to work with Kim to help regain a sense of wholeness through dialogue and negotiation.

The account is a powerful endorsement of the Burford NDU model to enable a dramatic shift in practitioner's thinking, feeling and behaviour. Those two cues 'How is the person feeling?' and 'How do I feel about the person?' seem on the surface so simple, so obvious and yet emerge as profound. The whole account reminds us that practice is not about doing things to patients but working with people – the human-human encounter.

Note also the role of guided reflection that enables Helen to become reflective in and on her practice, enabling her to become more focused and assertive in her holistic role with others. Note also the pattern of dialogue wherein I simply prod the dialogue onwards as Helen uses the dialogue to reflect on emerging issues and work things out to gain insight.

INVITATION TO DIALOGUE

The original Burford NDU model book published in 1994 was a reflection of its commitment to share its practice development to a wider audience. It also did this through its national teaching and visitor programme. This revised book is an extension of that commitment, an invitation to dialogue.

[To facilitate dialogue....

Wiley Blackwell has established a website.... (or through ICoP).]

NOTES

1 In *Becoming a Reflective Practitioner* (sixth edition) (Johns 2022) I set out my perception of the Reflective Curriculum (chapter 14) that grew out of my lecturer-practitioner role at Burford. Various chapters in this book expand upon appreciating and developing the reflective/holistic curriculum.

2 Leadership is not a given. It requires extensive development. Realising the significance of leadership I established the MSc Leadership in Health care programme grounded in leadership values and reflective practice. The students were required to construct a reflexive narrative of becoming the leader they desired to become. An analysis of more than a 100 narratives illuminated the barriers of realising desired leadership within their Transactional Organisations. See Johns C (2016) *Mindful Leadership*. Palgrave, London.

3 Helen's account is constructed from notes recorded from guided reflection session. The sessions were recorded to give Helen a record of dialogue as a secondary means of reflection and reminder to take action. Each subsequent session began with a review of the previous session and building on it reflexively. Constructing a reflexive narrative of guided reflection dialogue is extremely valuable in constructing a personal developmental portfolio.

REFERENCES

Graham J, Green M, and Stone S (1999) 'IT' has made a difference, hasn't it? *International Journal of Human Caring* 3(2); 39–46.

Johns C (1991) The Buford nursing development unit holistic model of nursing practice. *Journal of Advanced Nursing* 16; 1090–8.

Johns C (1994) Constructing the NBNDU model. In *The Buford NDU model: caring in practice* (Ed. C Johns) Blackwell Science, Oxford, p20–60.

Johns C (2022) *Becoming a reflective practitioner (sixth edition)* Wiley Blackwell, Oxford.

MacKintosh C (1998) Reflection: a flawed strategy for the nursing profession. *Nurse Education Today* 18; 553–7.

O'Brien B and Pope J (1994) Julia Farr centre nursing development unit: a model for practice. In *The Buford NDU model: caring in practice* (Ed. C Johns) Blackwell Science, Oxford, p187–208.

Watson J (1990) Caring knowledge and informed moral passion. *Advances in Nursing Science* 13(1); 15–24.

Wilber K (1998) *The eye of the spirit: an integral vision for a world gone slightly mad*. Shambhala, Boston.

Burford NDU Model Documentation

APPENDIX 1

Burford Community Hospital and Nursing Development Unit

Person narrative – personal data

Person .... D.o.b..............................

Wishes to be called ....

Single/married/widowed/ other

Address of usual residence: ....

....

Telephone: ....

Family/others at this residence: ....

Next of kin: ....

Address: ....

Tel numbers (h).............................. (m).......................... (w)..

Significant other(s): ....

Religious status: ....

Allergies	Subsequent admissions	
	Date	Reason
Past medical history		

GP	Tel:	Primary nurse

Burford Community Hospital and Nursing Development Unit

Narrative Assessment Cues:

Core question: 'What information do I need to be able to nurse this person?'

	Cue questions	
	Who is this person?	
	What health event brings this person into hospital?	
	How is this person feeling?	
	How has this event affected their usual life-pattern and roles?	
	How do I feel about this person?	
	How can I help this person?	
	What is important for this person to make their stay in hospital comfortable?	
	What support does this person have in life?	
	How does this person view the future for themselves and others?	

Burford Community Hospital and Nursing Development Unit

Person Narrative – information on admission	
Date	

Person: Primary nurse:

Date of admission

Burford Community Hospital and Nursing Development Unit

Person Narrative – Special Intervention Sheet

Patient Primary nurse

Burford Community Hospital and Nursing Development Unit

Person Narrative – continuation page

Date	Time	Prob no.	Evaluation/ planning/ progress	Sig.

Name P/N

Burford Community Hospital and Nursing Development Unit

Person narrative – Discharge planning
Patient P/N

Referred agencies	Contact	Referred agencies	Contact

Burford Community Hospital and Nursing Development Unit

Discharge Standard Protocol

Standard: Discharge is managed to maximise patient and carer ability to cope	
Protocol for key actions for primary nurses	
1	Primary nurse writes a summarised care plan where community nursing is required.
2	Primary nurse ensures all other workers are cognisant with the preparations for discharge.
3	Primary nurse identifies key worker(s) for continued care of the person. This will normally be either the home care organiser or district nurse.
4	The key worker should visit the patient at least 7 days prior to envisaged date for discharge to discuss future care arrangements with the primary nurse.
5	Primary nurse decides to instigate a home visit. When this is decided he/she is responsible for coordinating appropriate health care/social care workers to effectively achieve the standard.
6	Primary nurse informs patient/ carer(s) of likely discharge date at earliest possible time and confirms date as soon as possible.
7	Primary nurse confirms that the GP has discharged the patient from medical treatment necessitating hospital management.
8	Primary nurse informs family/ carer of rights to travel costs.
9	Primary nurse ensures that both patient and carer(s) accept the discharge plan
Notes This protocol negotiated and agreed by primary nurses following consultation with other health care workers involved in hospital and community care of patients and families.	

Burford Community Hospital and Nursing Development Unit

APPENDIX 2

Person narrative – care plan
Name: Reg Simpson

page
P/N: Lyn

Date	No.	Problem/need	Goal	Action	sig	Date resolved or plan altered
6/11	1	Reg says he's not managing well [SI sheet]	Explore and secure support for the future	Early dialogue with daughters and Discharge plan	cj	
6/11	2	Difficulty and anxiety with sleep	Improve his satisfaction with sleep	Use VAS sleep scale to monitor	cj	
6/11	3	Poor appetite – loss of taste/weight loss	Improve as possible	Discuss with cook and with daughters to identify favourite foods/drinks	cj	
6/11	4	Increasing loss of mobility	Improve as possible	Monitor/referral to physiotherapist	cj	
6/11	5	Fragile skin (prone to breakdown)	Prevent breakdown	Monitor daily + pressure relieving aids	cj	
6/11	6	Catheter in-situ	Maintain good hygiene	Self-care + catheter care as protocol as necessary	cj	
6/11	7	Prone to constipation	Use bowel chart to monitor	Increase fibre in diet? Improve mobility (see problem 3) Medication?	cj	
6/11	8	Self-care?	Reach potential for discharge	Monitor help required with him on a daily basis	cj	
6/11	9	Maintain lifestyle		Arrange delivery of Guardian newspaper Day care	cj	

Notes: These 'problems' overlap within an overall pattern of need stemming from Reg's statement – "I'm not managing well". The goals and planning are indeterministic at this initial stage.

Holistic Practice in Healthcare: The Burford NDU Person-centred Model, Second Edition. Edited by Christopher Johns.

Model for Structured Reflection 18th Edition (Johns 2022)

APPENDIX 3

Preparatory phase – Bring the mind home

Descriptive phase – Write a description of an experience [Dialogical movement 1]

Reflective phase cues [Dialogical movement 2]

What is significant to reflect on?

Why did I respond as I did?

Did I respond in tune with my vision?

Did I respond effectively in terms of consequences?

Did my feelings and attitudes influence me?

Did past experiences influence me?

Did I respond ethically for the best?

Anticipatory phase –

Given a similar situation, how could I respond more effectively, for the best and in tune with my vision?

Am I able to respond as envisaged?

Consider:

Am I skilful and knowledgeable enough to respond differently?

Am I powerful enough to respond differently?

Do I have the right attitude?

Am I poised enough to respond differently?

Insightful phase – What tentative insights do I draw from this experience?

Deepening insights phase

How has extant theory/ideas inform and deepen my insights? [Dialogical level 3]

How has guidance deepen my insights? [Dialogical movement 4]

How do I now feel about the experience?

Representation phase [Dialogical movement 5]

How can I communicate my insights most effectively in written/performance format?

Holistic Practice in Healthcare: The Burford NDU Person-centred Model, Second Edition. Edited by Christopher Johns.

REFERENCE

Johns C (2022) Engaging the reflective spiral: the second dialogical movement. In *Becoming a reflective practitioner* (sixth edition) Wiley Blackwell, Oxford. (chapter 4, pp. 36–51, Table 4.1).

Index

Page numbers in *italic* indicate figures; page numbers in **bold** indicate boxes or tables. Page numbers followed by 'n' refer to footnotes.

Holistic Practice in Healthcare: The Burford NDU Person-centred Model, Second Edition. Edited by Christopher Johns.

Printed and bound by CPI Group (UK) Ltd, Croydon, CR0 4YY
19/07/2023
03237796-0001